NEW LABOUR'S STATE OF HEALTH

For Leah, Josh and Tracey

New Labour's State of Health
Political Economy, Public Policy and the NHS

CALUM PATON
Keele University, UK

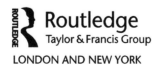

Routledge
Taylor & Francis Group

LONDON AND NEW YORK

First published 2006 by Ashgate Publishing

Published 2016 by Routledge
2 Park Square, Milton Park, Abingdon, Oxon OX14 4RN
711 Third Avenue, New York, NY 10017, USA

Routledge is an imprint of the Taylor & Francis Group, an informa business

British Library Cataloguing in Publication Data
Paton, Calum R., 1956-
  New Labour's state of health : political economy, public
  policy and the NHS
  1. Medical policy - Great Britain 2. National health
  services - Great Britain 3. Public health - Great Britain
  4. Medical economies - Great Britain
  I. Title
  362.1'0941
Library of Congress Cataloging-in-Publication Data
Paton, Calum, 1956-
  New labour's state of health : political economy, public policy and the NHS / by
Calum Paton.
       p. cm.
  Includes index.
  ISBN-13: 978-0-7546-4513-9
  ISBN-10: 0 7546-4513-4
  1. Medical policy--Great Britain. 2. National health services--Great Britain. 3.
Public health--Great Britian. 4. Medical economics--Great Britian. I. Title.

  RA395.G7P37 2006
  362.10941--dc22

                                                              2006020643

ISBN 9780754645139 (hbk)

Contents

Preface

This book has grown from theoretical work on political economy and health services, which I began to commit to paper three years ago, into a synthesis of political economy, public policy and New Labour's record, particularly as regards the NHS. As a political scientist, I construe 'New Labour's record' in terms of the political legitimacy and sustainability of its reforms and initiatives rather than (just) 'technical evaluation' of its various fragments of policy.

As well as being both a political theorist and specialist in health policy, I have recently been Chairman of one of the UK's largest NHS hospital Trusts, for five years up to the end of 2005 after being reappointed in 2004. The book has not therefore come out with indecent haste after my scribblings of 2003. That said, I think I have been motivated to complete it quickly in 2006 – with my academic concerns augmented by a desire more acute than usual to treat the worlds of theory and practice together!

I was often asked how I combined being a critical theorist and commentator with (what others construed, rightly or wrongly as) the role of an apparatchik. I tended to defuse the question by quoting the late Lord Hailsham, who – when asked how he combined being both judge and legislator/member of the executive – said, 'I'm sober as a judge but drunk as a Lord'!

More seriously, there's much to be sober about in today's NHS, the concept of which I endorse as fully as ever despite the culture which is being encouraged or allowed by politicians in England especially. At the theoretical level, the challenges of understanding how international political economy meets the 'domestic policy garbage can' to produce today's NHS are equally sobering.

I would like to thank – anonymously – many executives and staff I have met and worked with in the NHS, and who have (usually unconsciously) sharpened my understanding of how policy is implemented 'on the ground,' some of whom keep going in adverse conditions for altruistic reasons. And as ever I would like to thank those in academe who have challenged me in terms of my thesis.

Finally, my family as ever has contributed indirectly – but constantly – to this work. Combining theory with practice was (often) exhilarating – as the most tedious detail of policy in practice suddenly throws light on some theory supposedly worlds apart; or as a piece of grand theory suddenly lights up what seemed to be a confusing mess in practice. But it could also be frustrating. As ever, I'd like to thank Tracey for putting up with me when I became Victor Meldrew rather than Karl Marx, and to my children Leah and Josh who always cheered me up by showing me that both academe and the NHS should be put and kept in their place! Enoch Powell once said that his proudest achievement in life was winning a donkey derby. Seeing my daughter and son playing together in their 'first school' football team means more to me than getting to the bottom of New Labour's neuroses!

Acknowledgements

I would like to thank the *Journal of Health Economics, Policy and Law* (Cambridge University Press) for agreeing that text prepared for my article entitled, 'Choice in the English NHS: Visible Hand or Invisible Fist?' (to be published in early 2007), could be adapted and incorporated in Chapter 7 of this book. I would also like to thank *Hospital* (the journal of European hospital managers) for permission to adapt and incorporate a short article entitled 'Going Private' (Issue 2, 2006) within Chapter 6 of this book.

Introduction: Political Economy, Public Policy and New Labour

This book explains the influence of political economy upon public policy. It also illustrates, in theory and practice, how political economy interacts with other significant factors which help to explain public policy. It does this by examining health policy made and implemented by New Labour. It examines health policy under New Labour in its own right, but also in order to trace some general features both of New Labour's approach to government and of the policy process in modern Britain (especially England, in that much of the empirical material in Part 3 in particular is drawn, post-devolution, from England rather than the other parts of the UK).

Health policy has some special characteristics, based on New Labour's diagnosis of the NHS's problems both pre- and post-1997, but it also exemplifies in important respects the general approach to domestic policy of New Labour. This is not surprising. Just as the Conservative health reforms of the 1990s drew on approaches which were generic to the public sector as a whole, New Labour's public sector agenda contains themes applied to health but by no means unique to health. In a nutshell, general politics in health is more significant than the specific politics of health, although the public sector 'reform agenda' has had some pretty counter-intuitive and perverse effects when applied to health.

The title of the book deliberately has a triple reference. In reverse order: firstly, there is health (explored in detail in Part 3) – referring to how health services and health are or are not prospering under New Labour. Secondly, there is the state: Part 2 examines the role and nature of the state, public policy-making and implementation under New Labour government, with health policy as the main focus. Thirdly there is New Labour – and Part 1 uses strategy for health services to illustrate how the New Labour stance on political economy is the driver of the 'New Labour project'.

Political Economy

The subtitle points to my diagnosis of political economy as a major determining factor in explaining health policy. In Part 1, it is argued that health reflects general features of political economy, politics and policy which derive from the imperatives that a country such as Britain confronts when living in a regime of global capitalism. The manner of adapting to such a regime is not however mechanistically determined – and the strategies adopted by New Labour in England (and Labour elsewhere in

Britain) may differ from that in other countries. At the most general level, some questions must be asked, in order to set British or specifically English policy in context.

The most basic difference between countries is whether or not the private sector or public sector predominates in (especially) financing but also providing healthcare. If (as I have argued elsewhere (Paton, 2001)) capitalism benefits from an active role of the state in public healthcare as with the British National Health Service (NHS) despite the orthodox or naïve view that the 'capitalist state' is the minimalist state, then why does the U.S. state not conform to this pattern? The answer is two-fold.

Firstly, private healthcare providers – but also, and especially, financiers (such as insurance companies and corporate Health Maintenance Organisations (Feachem et al, 2002)) – are a salient part of the capitalist economy. (The same is not true in the UK.) As a result, corporate influence of the private health sector upon the US state is significant, and tends to prohibit any comprehensive strategy to 'rationalise' through public control. This applies even if such control were not to be motivated by social reform (let alone socialism) but by the sort of 'capitalist rationality' which uses public health services as a parsimonious means of investing in the health of employees to the benefit of the capitalist economy. What is more, the fragmented nature of the US state (Paton, 1990) means that specific corporate strata and interests (such as health financiers and providers) bring direct, uncoordinated pressure to bear upon the state unlike in the UK. In the latter, such pressure may exist, but the central and centralising state has an active role in coordinating demands which is relatively absent in the US, given its policy process and legislative 'modus operandi'. In the US, the factors responsible for stalling the Clinton Plan for national health coverage in 1993-4 illustrate this well. (Mann and Ornstein, Eds, 1995). In particular, we can note the 'micro-pluralism' which sees increasingly specialised and narrow interests interacting with a Congress which is ever-more decentralised as regards domestic policy-making.

Secondly, private corporations in the US economy as a whole use health benefits (insurance and coverage) as a 'perk' – a tool for recruitment and retention of the 'scarce and skilled', whether white or blue collar – to an increasingly old-fashioned and blurred dividing-line. The opposite applies too: the 'plentiful and unskilled' are the ones without insurance. There is a 'path dependency' in policy which makes it difficult to break out of this approach and create new policy with new incentives. In the language of Part 2 of this book, institutional bias in making public policy (behaviour patterns created or encouraged by political structures) interacts with political economy to create incentives (for corporations as well as policy-makers) which are difficult to replace with a new 'rational' strategy.

Another question concerns the nature of a socialised healthcare system in a capitalist society. If a public NHS co-exists with the 'capitalist state', then what constraints does this put upon such an NHS? What are the tendencies in financing (i.e. by which types of taxpayer? how generously?), provision (i.e. which services for whom?) and employment (of whom? under what conditions?) How have changing regimes in political economy affected health services? Is there such a thing as a 'third way' between Keynesian social democracy and Thatcherism? These factors are explored in Part 1 of this book. Here it should be noted that New Labour, while it has dropped the glib rhetoric of the 'Third Way' (Giddens, 1998; Paton, 2000), has made 'public service reform' the litmus-test of both its record and its distinctiveness, in it third term after the general election of 2005 – building on markers put down in its second term, especially in education and health (the 'core' of the publicly-funded welfare state in the twenty-first century.) If this reform is not just the Thatcherism which Lady Thatcher did not dare attempt twenty years earlier, we must ask: how does 'social investment' New Labour-style differ from what Marxists, writing in the 1970s (O'Connor, 1973; Gough, 1979; Navarro, 1978) would have expected the capitalist state to do? I believe it does not. And if it does not, then the ideologists of the 'third way' such as Giddens have huffed and puffed to disguise the hollowness of their claims.

Public Policy

Part 2 examines the main 'causal factors' explaining public policy, and explains how political economy interacts with other factors. There is thus an engagement with the general literature from political science about the public policy process. A hierarchy of factors which are useful in explaining public policy is presented. The manner in which these factors interact is clearly important in explaining policy, but arguably even more so in explaining the manner in which it is implemented. This is especially true when different 'streams' of policy co-exist in tension or even conflict, and both public management and political economy require solutions of a particular sort.

To illustrate, building on the considerations introduced above: the national and international political economy confronting a country might seem to call for welfare and health policy of a particular sort (see Part 1 below). We might call this the 'rational strategy' for a government to pursue (ignoring for now the complications of the term 'rationality' in social science.) This is not intended to be overly 'functionalist' (implying that, 'cometh the need, cometh the policy'). Nor is it intended to suggest, even less plausibly, an 'evolutionist' approach to understanding policy (John, 1999). This approach is based on an analogy with evolution in natural science, yet forgets that the political 'environment' to which policies allegedly have to be 'adapted' is also changeable by human agency; and that therefore the approach is either tautologous or vacuous.

Instead, attributing rationality to government requires an assumption of instrumentalism (i.e. we have to identify who devises 'what' and acts 'how' in pursuit of ends, rather than just assuming that it 'happens.') An assumption of rationality may be misleading or at least requiring severe qualification (see Part 2). It is argued in Part 2 however that (in health at least) government is aware of the need for a comprehensive strategy to meet economic, social and political needs. Unfortunately for the coherence of policy, it is left to 'meso'-level intermediaries, and late in the day to boot, to seek to coordinate policy.

In health for example, a government operating in the age of globalisation might see advantages in a national health service which sought to combine a number of characteristics – investing in the health of productive workers employed in those economic 'niches' giving the country comparative advantage; ensuring that pivotal strata and voters to whom the health issue was salient were satisfied with the health service; and protecting the poor, either in the name of equity or in order to promote social and political stability. Such a complex agenda will likely require the most careful and 'rational' tailoring of public resources in a highly efficient manner to make such multiple aims compatible (if indeed such is possible). In a nutshell, the strategy requires appropriate policies; an adequate coordination of policies to make them consistent and avoid perverse outcomes through perverse or clashing incentives; and effective implementation.

Incoherent policy-making or perverse effects in implementation are likely to make the system politically or economically untenable (even if we wish to avoid a word such as dysfunctional) – as a result of one or more of such aims not being adequately met. What, then, if the effect of political structure or culture upon public policy pulls in a different direction to that of the 'rational executive's' agenda? Or what if 'post-modern' policy comes out of the 'garbage-can' containing transient and incoherent items, rather than the ivory tower manned by boffins rationally tailoring means to ends in the 'public interest.'?

To make it sound less academic: how can the New Labour machine, staffed by legislators and advisers characterised by 'pledge card policy, tick-box implementation and sound bite communication' – with lofty aspirations in inverse proportion to both policy coherence and the modern political attention span – deliver? What does health policy tell us about this? Is New Labour, despite its wads of extra pounds for the NHS, about to snatch defeat from the jaws of victory? This is perfectly possible on current indications: Labour is demanding more productivity in the NHS yet incurring huge costs both through the very 'market mechanisms' to which it is a late convert and through the co-existence of contradictory policies – all of which are expensive. It is more than a straw in the wind that, since Christmas 2005, the English media have been highlighting the co-existence of record revenue for the NHS (approaching £90 billion by 2006) and record financial deficits and 'denials of care' to save money. Yet the cost of contradictory policy is about three times the national deficit (Paton, 2006e). It is not rocket science to 'sort this out', and show that a state-funded NHS can prosper. Yet New Labour's confused policy is ironically discrediting the state model.

Assuming it is not too late and that the state (NHS) model is not doomed as a result of incompetence, what are the mechanisms by which different policy streams, or rather waves, can be made to flow in the same direction of the direction of the overall aims? And what does this tell us about how tightly the public sector has to be centrally controlled? That is, despite the cyclical and recently-revived rhetoric of devolution and local control (never mind the revived aspiration of a healthcare market which seemingly has New Labour seeking to 'out-macho' the ghost of

Thatcher), is central control inevitable and even desirable (or at least acceptable in the absence of legitimate regional institutions)?

Is the aspiration of 'the new market' in the NHS undermined firstly by 'policy overload' (in part occasioned by a 'post-modern' profusion of incoherent policy streams) and secondly by the need to use the coordinating (and therefore centralising) power of the state and its 'meso'-level agencies to rationalise this policy overload.? Just as the Tory internal market's 'managed competition' (always a gloss on a messy reality) was an oxymoron (lapsing into management or market but not both (Paton et al, 1998), is New Labour's 'regulated market' equally unstable? And does this apply only to health or to the 'big idea' of New Labour's second and third terms across the public sector as a whole? Part 2 seeks to answer these questions.

Health Policy

In Part 3, an examination of the conundrums of recent health policy analyses policy 'on the ground' in England but also elucidates further some of the arguments in Part 2, in illustrating the role of the state.

This closer examination of health policy allows us to see the government's intentions more clearly – for the simple reason that it is the main area of public policy where central government not only controls policy-making but also is responsible for the provision of most of the services (despite some of the prevailing rhetoric.) We can see that New Labour is highly sensitive to how 'atypical' the NHS is in today's world (where state control is likely to be depicted as 'old-fashioned, bureaucratic, nationalised industry'), which colours, or rather waters down, its defence of the public approach to running health services.

This explains the obsession of Secretaries of State such as Alan Milburn (Health, 1999 to 2003) with denying that they are 'Stalinists': every half-baked reform and re-organisation since 1999 has been born from this political symbolism rather than from a diagnosis of health-sector need. Yet in reality, and with concealed irony (New Labour doesn't do irony): by dismantling planning institutions at the middle level between state and locality (so-called 'meso institutions'), or rather deepening the Tories' dismantling, New Labour has left central government as the primary lever-puller. In 2006, in the new NHS where the health Trust 'regulator' (not 'Offsick' but Monitor!) is regulating Foundation Trusts (and aspirants i.e. all hospital Trusts) in a rhetorical environment of devolution, 'patient choice' and private financing, central direction is nevertheless stronger than ever. Yet to detect this, one has to have a nose for the political irony whereby 'all is not as it seems' (for the invisible fist of power as well as the visible hand of the 'new regulation'), as well as an understanding of recent history and a healthy scepticism. The search for what's really happening has to be a more painstaking one than in the early 1990s when the Tories were steaming through the public sector, for there is no sense of metaphysical doubt on the part of New Labour even in off-the-record briefings or off-the-cuff remarks. For New Labour Ministers, in their more po-faced incarnation, make at least one mistake the

Conservatives did not make in the 1990s as regards health reform – they believe their own rhetoric. Not for them Kenneth Clarke's insouciance as regards his own government's 'market reforms' in the NHS in 1990, when he said, 'It's my opponents who talk of markets, not me'!

Centralism is dead; long live centralism. If New Labour was not so terrified of the power of right-wing and pro-market ideology (or rather the power of the tabloids to invoke the ghost of Old Labour past), this might not be all a bad thing. If 'centralism' meant planning of services to meet public objectives by 'meso level' institutions such as regional health authorities, then it would only be the public sector analogue of what large private corporations use to meet private objectives. Yet New Labour dare not invoke 'Stalinist' words such as planning, even when they are meat and drink to private sector consultancies like McKinsey's, on the one hand, and corporations such as Sainsbury's, on the other.

As a result, there is in the NHS an absence of effective meso-level institutions (intermediaries between the central state and those local agencies responsible for providing actual services), which means that central government has to issue disjointed commands down different vertical 'silos' of the Department of Health. This is centralism with 'knobs on', in which the left hand's bells doesn't know which tune the right hand's whistles are blowing. Surprise, surprise ... the government is ridiculed for 'command and control' (by those same newspapers which have Mr. Milburn and his successors for breakfast, as they pick up on the groans of both clinicians and managers in the NHS who are sick both of 'managing to targets' and of seeing services 'slashed and burned' to prepare their Trust for the 'new market' – services recently developed to meet government targets, at that!). And crucially, to add another layer of irony, such command is rendered less susceptible to control – as a result of those cumbersome and counter-productive 'devolved institutions' at the local level (eg Primary Care Trusts and Foundation Trusts.) New Labour argues that it has abolished 'command and control' (with echoes of the quickly-discredited 'Third Way') but in fact it has deepened the command state while disabling the control state (yet still requiring it – hence the tortuous 'backdoor' means of planning the health service discussed below in Part 3).

And so ...New Labour's State of Health ...

New Labour is obsessed with appearing 'relevant' in the age of global capitalism – but not by clipping the state's wings. The New Labour state is a bossy and priggish state, yet quite amateurish in its statecraft. In this it is actually very Old Labour – confident when wearing the Tories' clothes on the battlefield, yet tentative in leading, as opposed to following, in economic and domestic policy. Perhaps we can call it the 'boy scout state', although there are plenty girl scouts around too with a pious zeal to organise society.

And these modern Fabians relish micro management of and in the public services. As well as New Labour's 'new market', we have both micro-management by politicians linked to the modern industry known as 'risk management' and the hierarchies required to run and police it on a scale undreamt of in the 1990s. We see this in the universities and wider education sector on a similar scale. Yet it is debatable how much this actually helps: the paradox of 'governance' is that it works when you don't need it (i.e. when those being governed are both doing the right thing and reporting it to their governors) and rarely works when you do need it (i.e. when executives are not 'telling their governors what they don't know') The most perfectly structured assurance system requires people to fill the structures with the right information. More importantly, the uneasy combination of markets and hierarchy suits New Labour's temperament (it has given up on planning, but is peopled by former Leftists with itchy fingers) yet may often provide the 'worst of both worlds' (of the market and hierarchy) rather than the best of both as the more naïve versions of the 'third way' would have it.

Micro-management is much more present today than in 1948, despite the superficial language of 'devolution' from the central state and central government to other actors, and the rhetoric of a state (borrowed from both American management gurus and John Major in the early 1990s) which 'steers but does not row.' (Osborne and Gaebler, 1993) To criticise micro-management is not to criticise state responsibility for financing and providing healthcare. To its credit, Britain has sought a different approach to 'investing in health' from that found in the USA, for example – relying broadly upon public financing via the NHS to seek to placate 'middle Britain, whereas the US continues to eschew public financing of mainstream healthcare. In this respect, New Labour is more like Old Labour than in other policy areas. Prime Minister Blair was thus right, in the Foreword to the NHS Plan of July 2000, to describe the NHS as the greatest act of modernisation undertaken by a Labour government (Blair, 2000).

The trouble is that, rather than boast unequivocally of this stance, New Labour is Janus-faced. While it wants the credit from its own backbenchers and core support for this stance, it is embarrassed by it when socialising and 'policy wonking' in its newer haunts on the Right. (See next paragraph.) As a result, it maintains the public NHS surreptitiously, while disabling the 'meso-level' planning mechanisms which such a service needs to be governed and coordinated effectively (see Part 3 of this book.) New Labour's amateurish but itchy fingers as regard 'NHS reform' have prioritised disparate, conflicting and perpetual policy initiatives – to prove its 'modern' and 'market' credentials to the media – over coherent governance and management of the service. As a result, the NHS has received much new money but has been politically destabilised at the same time, with some of the new money used to the good but much of it frittered and wasted through: anarchic commissioning (purchasing) arrangements; poor value-for-money in both public/private 'partnerships' and out-sourcing; and new contracts for doctors and (other) employees which have belied the tough rhetoric (see Part 3's elucidation of the factors which explain the use of the new money.) This is a spectacular own goal.

And defences of public planning (which at its best is less bureaucratic than both market and 'micro-managing' alternatives) do Labour no good within the portals of its newer haunts – the think-tanks of the market (such as Reform) and of the Right (such as the Centre for a New Europe); the newspapers and journals for whom any publicly-planned service is a 'Stalinist' dinosaur; and the domains of those transatlantic 'neo-conservative' commentators, such as Irwin Stelzer (2006), with views would have seemed old-fashioned fifty years ago yet which have 'come around again' in the guise of modernism. It is these commentators who laud Blair's international neo-conservatism yet bemoan the cobwebs of his reluctant Labourism at home – uneasy bedfellows such as Stephen Pollard, official biographer of David Blunkett. New Labour has ridden a tiger from which it now cannot easily dismount.

Factions which are variously pro-globalisation of the most capitalist hue, neo-conservative and both penetrated to the heart of Tony Blair's thinking, and 'gelled' with his desire to attack the 'forces of conservatism' (interestingly, a phrase he used with the doctors much in mind) (Blair, 1999; Hyman, 2005, p 89-92). Blair allegedly remarked, on foreign policy, "Neoconservatism is merely progressive politics by another name" (Stelzer, *op.cit*) – a remark which shows his peculiar understanding of the term 'progressive', as well as his ignorance of the origins and beliefs of the current 'neo-cons.'

Whether Brown has a different approach is another question. Of the perpetual 'boy scout' tinkering with public sector reform, he is less guilty. Yet it was his own 'target-itis' driven from the Treasury, burdening the NHS with a regime which led in turn to senior health executives 'managing to target' rather than managing the service, which led to Milburn's 'recantation' of this approach, and his search – amateurish but possibly sincere – for an alternative 'consumerist' approach. Brown has been the godfather of the PFI, New Labour-style, with the Treasury and wider government absorbing, indeed embodying, the private interests and individuals who benefit from that approach. Brown and Milburn may have been political enemies, but they have been Tweedledee and Tweedledum in terms of domestic policy.

In domestic policy, New Labour has wanted to paw and finger all the trendy toys from the New Right nursery – albeit in even more bureaucratised form than witnessed under the centralising Tories of the 1990s. As well as the 'purchaser/provider split', 'managed choice', patient vouchers and so on, this includes the discredited Private Finance Initiative (PFI) (Paton, 2006a), invented by Norman Lamont, Tory Chancellor of the Exchequer, at the beginning of the 1990s and subsequently disowned by him at least as far as health is concerned. The Conservative party leader elected at the end of 2005, David Cameron, went further in hinting that the PFI was yesterday's policy – and at the beginning of 2006, Secretary of State for Health Patricia Hewitt (archetypal New Labour Minister with a radical past and Blairite present) was beginning to worry about the inflexibility and cost of the PFI in the light of the structural deficit confronting the English acute hospital sector (see Part 3). As ever, if you borrow the nasty capitalists' policy and ignore the warnings from both left and right, neither of the latter will support you when the reckoning comes. This is more Very Old Labour – when Prime Minister Ramsay Macdonald was the 'fall guy' in the 1930s, eventually pushed out by the enemies he had cuddled up to – than New Labour (if the latter is supposed to mean 'street-wise capitalism-lite'.) To be dished by the Tories from the left, allowing Cameron's Tory Party to represent Disraeli as against the stern Gladstonian Brown (with his Kirkcaldy kirk-based socialism now replaced by the philosophy of Kirkcaldy's Adam Smith), is actually an impressive error!

As well as flexing its Thatcherite muscles with markets and neologistic, hybrid market mechanisms in the public sector, New Labour has sought to spin itself as different and demonstrate its **post**-Thatcherite modernity by emphasizing terms such as 'governance' and 'networks'. The idea is that both traditional public administration, on the one hand, and laisser-faire (or markets – not the same thing), on the other hand, are old hat; and that there is a 'third way' (despite the demise into ridicule of the term itself) through which new forms of mobilisation and action in the economy can be characterised. For about two decades now, in political science, the term 'governance', as opposed to government, has been a trendy way to characterise the alleged complexity (or public/private mutual embeddedness) of modern government. The implication is that the 'official' state, both central and local, is only one part of a jigsaw which must be put together if action is either to occur in practice or to be explained by the theorist.

I am suspicious of the salience of this concept, at the very least in the field of British health policy. 'Governance' is a gerundive word, supposedly pointing to the open-ended and pluralistic structure of policy making, which is 'work in progress' rather than tablets of stone from the government. To that extent it loosely reflects a kind of kitchen-sink post-modernism applied to the field of public policy. As a modest metaphor with much to be modest about (apologies to Churchill), it can be borne. But the work in political science on 'governance' through networks is not noteworthy for its explanatory value. (Dowding, 1995; 2001). And New Labour's translation of its vision into an original strategy or blueprint is conspicuous by its absence.

After nearly ten years of New Labour government, the third way has collapsed in practice as well as in theory. We are discovering that, after all, there is something distinctive about the public sector (as against the 1990s Tory view that all it required were private sector ethos and techniques, and the New Labour 'touchy feely' version of the same) We are also discovering that the private sector, in turn, is pretty immune to New Labour's wishful thinking (Blair, 1996) as to its transformation into a brave new world of partnerships and collaboration.

In the English health sector, we are re-learning that you cannot have both planning and markets ('managed markets', the Tories had called it in the 1990s) without one collapsing into the other. When asked in 2003 how New Labour's health reforms differed from the Tories' market reforms in the 1990s, Paul Corrigan, the political adviser to the Secretary of State for Health said, "they bottled out; we're not going to." (Presentation at Department of Health). Brave new world, indeed. But, by 2006, two Secretaries of State later, history was repeating itself, somewhat farcically (see Part 3), only one decade after the lesson had been learned the first time around: however much bottle you have, a planned or managed market in a public health care system is an oxymoron. Professor Ray Robinson, a respected health policy analyst who had been prepared to work with the concept, argued in September 2003 at a Judge Institute conference in Cambridge that he had come belatedly to believe that you could have a planned NHS or a market system, but not both.

The key question, then, is which way Labour – and the country as a whole – eventually 'turns', on health policy. This 'turn' will not be from a loss of 'bottle', but because of the analytical and therefore (eventual) political incoherence of the 'third way.'

A Comparative Note

Briefly comparing New Labour's healthcare state with the previous Conservative government's 'reformed NHS' in the 1990s, as done in Part 3 of this book, has two advantages – firstly, we can keep recent reforms in perspective; and secondly, we can discern any significant features of British public policy-making and implementation (i.e. the 'policy process') which may be common to both eras, or part of a trend.

It might be considered useful to set New Labour's health reforms (reality, not rhetoric) in a comparative European context. This is however done only at the most general level in this book, at the end of Part 3, as the focus is upon linking different levels of political explanation (from political economy at one extreme to the messy politics of implementation, at the other). To do this for other countries requires separate, detailed studies, which have been undertaken elsewhere (Paton et al, 2000). Whether or not New Labour's 'direction of travel' is typical or atypical is considered briefly but from the viewpoint of the political explanation of policy, not the internal analytics of health policy. Most European comparative health policy analysis is a 'politics-free zone' (or at least features politics as an inert backdrop) within which different reform programmes are 'rationally' compared. (Saltman et al, 2002) Such exercises may be useful in classifying and codifying systems (although there should be a major health warning around both perceived similarities – such as the 'purchaser/provider split' – and also perceived differences – such as 'national health services' versus 'social insurance.) They offer however neither a normative choice among alternatives nor a prognosis for the future. Studies which do this moreover (for example the WHO's World Health Reports (2000; 2006), with their criteria for 'good' systems, or macro-economic studies such as those of the OECD which analyse 'macro productivity') are not capable of linking cause and effect. Advocacy of health sector reform is, if not an evidence-free zone, one characterised by 'lies, damned lies and comparative evidence.'

Somewhat against the spirit of the age, therefore, this book implicitly suggests that 'internal comparison' of policies, that is longitudinal case studies, provide the best route to understanding both change and the possibilities for improvement. Inter-country comparison has been responsible for many static studies and dead-ends because of 'political naivety' – ideas and structures may be 'transplanted' from one system to another (eg. the Health Maintenance Organisation) without adequate reference to context, culture and prevailing structures. As long as there is willingness to set objectives for the health care system (both ethical and economic), to start with a judgement as to the best arrangements for realising these and to be honest in appraising success or otherwise, the modern morbidity of 'comparison-itis' (with its side-effect of rapidly spreading international consultants) can be minimised.

It should at once be admitted that 'judgement' incorporates a liberal understanding of the international history of health care systems. For example, what is a national health service (NHS) seeking that could not be found in either the USA or central Europe? And do the 'economic facts' imply that the NHS model is no longer capable of tackling productivity issues, for example? These questions should not be ducked, and are addressed in Part 3 in exploring 'where the money has gone.' But they should not be answered in a vacuum; nor should today's moral panics be allowed to destroy yesterday's achievements which may still hold currency for tomorrow's goals.

A publicly-planned NHS may have the capacity to achieve both equity and economy on a scale which other types of healthcare system cannot, including the 'modern' objectives of integrated care for the patients across organisational boundaries. If the NHS is not currently doing so, it is important not to 'throw the baby out with the bathwater', especially if present shortcomings are not explained (only) by inadequate incentives but also by confused incentives and clashing policy 'streams.' (see Part 3) This is especially true when other countries are dismantling the sorts of healthcare systems which English reform is aping. Comparison is valuable after all …but with a focussed purpose – as a servant not master.

PART 1
Political Economy

Chapter 1

Political Economy: Economic Regimes, Political Regimes and Political Economy in Britain

Changing Regime

In a nutshell, the move from the era of 'Keynesian' social democracy to our 'post-Fordist capitalist era of today is the move from an era when redistribution was politically feasible but increasingly impossible economically – to an era when redistribution is economically viable but politically difficult. In the first era of 'Fordism' – with mass production, mass consumption and mass welfare – redistribution was based on 'left-of-centre' electoral and political majorities but increasingly difficult economically. If the 'majority working class' voted itself benefits, the profit margin was squeezed and both Marxist left (Glyn and Sutcliffe, 1972) and monetarist Right (Bacon and Eltis, 1976) agreed that, in this environment, 'centrist' social democracy was untenable.

In the second era, the class structure of 'post-Fordism' was different – composed of separate strata, based on economic niches in both national and international economies, with a few a lot better-off; most a little better-off while working a lot harder; and the 'underclass' (about 10-20%) worse-off and working in unskilled jobs or not at all. In this era, redistribution also meant something different: it was limited to the 'underclass', as the political majority was aspirant and 'right-of-centre' (Galbraith, 1992) and was not seeking 'social benefit' (except for state-funded subsidies to middle-class purchases, such as houses, or what were still universal services such as health and education). Initially, while limited redistribution was economically possible (new wealth and less ambition for the redistribution), it was politically infeasible during the Thatcherite high noon, the 'loadsamoney' 1980s when the devil took the hindmost.

Later however there were both economic and social reasons for doing something about the embarrassing reminder that 'post-Fordism' had a weak underbelly. So redistribution meant 'tidying up the bottom of the heap' or taking the ' 10-20 %' out of poverty and seeking to 'count in' the underclass to the new society of 'permanent revolutionary consumerism', at whatever menial level. Shorn of its rhetoric, the latter was the essence of the New Labour project (hence stealth taxes, minimum wage and tax credits) – to sanitise the Thatcherite dung-heap of its smell without radically altering the structure! In fairness, it has succeeded – although such success is equivocal for a party of the left, in that – once again – Labour's historic mission has translated in practice into making capitalism safe and socially acceptable.

The Origins of Crisis

Incentives for capitalists to invest had diminished as the 1970s moved to 'crisis'. 'Left-of-centre politics' had dominated both Labour and Conservative governments after the 'post-war settlement', from the 1950s to the 1970s. The 'Butskellism' of the 1950s and 1960s (named after the Conservatives Rab Butler and Labour's Hugh Gaitskell (Williams, 1979)) had been followed by Premier Edward Heath's 1972 'U-turn', under pressure from trade unions, which seemed to re-affirm centrism. Social democracy was still (just) viable in terms of electoral behaviour – hence the Labour victories in 1974, albeit with reduced percentages of the vote by comparison with the 1960s.

Things were beginning to fall apart, however; the centre was not holding very well. Britain seemed to be 'against itself' (Beer, 1982), with the centrist orthodoxy challenged from both the left and industrial strong-arming (not the same thing) in the Labour party; and, from 1975 onwards, by a resurgent monetarist right in the Conservative party. It was in other words the 'last chance saloon' for the semi-planned economy, with prices and incomes policies as part of a general political settlement (the trade unions, in Harold Macmillan's phrase, had "never had it so good" but could only finally see that more than two decades later, when the Thatcher 'economic settlement' was confirmed by New Labour.) The electorate had seen, first, the Labour government's and, second, the Tories' industrial relations initiatives undermined by the trade unions; and the 1974 Labour victories were the last chance for a centrist social democracy which – given the climate of militancy – often looked like anything but.

This political regime was however also undermined by the decline of the economic regime. As the economic decline and 'crises' filtered through to political crises, an alternative regime in political economy was increasingly sought by both left and right. This in turn led to a political re-alignment based on an electoral realignment.

The politics of 'spending more' came to be replaced by the politics of 'taxing less', as the 'swing voters' from those strata of the working class undergoing 'embourgeoisement' (Goldthorpe et al, 1968) found that (variously) affluence, the prospect of affluence or the illusion of affluence meant a changed calculation as the costs and benefits of tax and spending. In the 1970s, higher wages had often been extorted by industrial muscle – superficially in the name of socialism but actually in the pursuit of sectional benefit. (Brian Abel-Smith, a health policy advisor to Barbara Castle, Health Secretary in the 1970s, had put it nicely in a Fabian pamphlet, "Socialism is about equality; trade-unionism is about differentials.") In the 1980s and 1990s, when Thatcherite economic policy and industrial reform ensured that relative affluence could only be earned not extorted, it was too late: acquiring the latest consumables for the family meant a treadmill from which it was too risky to jump – both for individuals and for classes, with the rise of globalisation and competitive threat to whole industries.

Implications of the New Regime for Health and Welfare

Lower taxes, given the downward pressure on wages in the world economy, became the means by which the middle and even worse-off strata sought a viable income (with more take hone-pay as a result of lower taxes 'outvoting' more social benefit except for those who derived unequivocal net benefit from the latter).

For health, this might have radical implications in theory. For those in work or part of the 'contented majority', why not 'pay as you go', or rather insure yourself, if public insurance or public taxation meant subsidy to the poorer – which was no longer politically necessary (as in the era of the left-of-centre majority). While politics and culture are thankfully never as simple as this, the moral from this possibility was not lost on New Labour. They knew the NHS had to justify every penny. And if it was to please the middle-classes and give them as much 'bang for the buck' for their taxes as insuring themselves privately would do while **also** redistributing to poor people and public health programmes, it would have to be hyper-efficient.

The question, then, was not : is the NHS more efficient than private alternatives. Of course it is. The question was: is it **so much more** efficient that it can fulfil a triple mission of pleasing 'middle England' (both health-wise and tax-wise), investing in the economy and reducing health inequalities. The jury is still out – although perhaps understandably it is the first two which have dominated in practice despite ambitions to reduce health inequalities which have not yet been realised. Even the NHS's 'target regime' has diluted the focus on inequalities (See Part 3).

After all, even if public provision is more efficient than private provision, it would still be possible for public services to be privately purchased by insured individuals and groups – the case has to be continually re-made for both public provision and public financing. Indeed New Labour has focussed on the latter, as it believes that private provision ' at the margin and more' may be more efficient.

Political economy's effects upon public policy may be exemplified by health policy as follows. Globalisation and further internationalisation of capital creates particular constraints for regimes of taxation and public expenditure. The provision of healthcare is a means of securing what the Marxist James O'Connor (1973), writing in the 1970s, called social investment as well as 'social expenses'. Investing in healthcare can be investment in the productive process (i.e. labour) and also investment in corporations to give them competitive advantage in the world economy. Either or both may involve the state in a central role. Some countries (such as the UK) use the state both to provide equitable health services and to prioritise health expenditures in line with economic needs.

This premise has a number of implications for an institution such as the National Health Service and for health policy more generally. Investing in the health of individuals or corporations can be carried out privately or through the state. In the United States it is primarily the former; in the UK the latter. If the state has a dominant role, it can be conceptualised as acting either on behalf of all society or on behalf of capital. The latter view is the traditional Marxist view, although it should be noted that it does not necessitate the 'vulgar Marxist' view which has the state as the executive committee of the bourgeoisie. The likelihood today is that, in statist health systems in capitalist society within a global capitalist world, the state will have to balance both roles.

The tensions here can be summed up as follows. Firstly, the international economy calls for low corporate tax, and possibly low personal tax. This in turn necessitates a restrictive regime of 'rationed' healthcare. Yet on the other hand, quite apart from investing in the health of workers to the benefit of the economy (or niches within the international economy), the state may develop a direct or indirect industrial policy to support native industries (whether native to Britain or to Europe), in the light of international competition. Clearly the medical technology and pharmaceutical industry are cases in point. From the viewpoint of government expenditure, it may be important to restrict access to new drugs from the public purse. Yet it may also be important to provide a welcoming home for multinational and national companies for the development of new products.

Secondly, there is also a tension between the classic egalitarian mission of the NHS as defined by socialists and social democrats, on the one hand, and economic investment using statist health services, on the other hand. Add to this the pressures from more virulent consumerism, on the one hand, and more active citizenship, on the other hand, and we can see how an institution such as the NHS becomes financially squeezed irrespective of its 'efficiency'. The question for the NHS is not, 'is it more efficient than alternative systems?'; the real question, again, is, 'is it so much more efficient than alternative systems that it can provide both a Fordist service for the mass of the population and also a post-Fordist service for economically privileged niches therein?'

In more concrete terms a variation of the above tension is expressed in the 'antithesis' of curative care and repair, on the one hand, and prevention and promotion on the other hand. Here we find conventional textbooks (eg Ham, 2004) giving a superficial impression of what a Marxist argument would be. The Marxist argument applied to British health services is often referred to through the writing of Navarro – in particular, his 1970s analysis of the National Health Service (*op. cit*). The NHS is caricatured as high technology medicine for the masses rather than a preventive socialist policy. The alleged rationale is to 'buy off' the masses. A related argument is that it is not complex technology which requires centralisation in health services, but centralisation for political reasons (barely explained) which leads to an emphasis on complex technology.

Both these related arguments are simply wrong. The idea that, in the socialist society, ordinary people will not want access to the most advanced technology is almost anti-diluvian in its naivety, and also deeply patronising. Next, there are 'neutral', planning-based reasons for centralisation and regionalisation of services which make Navarro's argument a caricature. But perhaps most importantly, there is a much more convincing Marxist case to be made about the role of the state in health services. It concerns, in Marxist terms, the extraction of surplus value in public services, to the benefit of the private economy (Paton, 1997).

Thirdly, political economy also affects the nature of employment in a service such as the NHS. There is much debate about whether post-Fordism and the change from the Keynesian National Welfare State to the post-Fordist economy directly affects the nature and organisation of welfare services. (There are of course debates about the validity of the construct of post-Fordism itself. I do not propose to engage with these here.) I argue below that it is misleading to imply that the organisation of the workforce (economy-wide) has immediate parallels for the organisation of the workforce in a service such as the NHS. It is more convincing to depict evolving employment in the NHS as exhibiting characteristics of neo-Fordism rather than post-Fordism. Neo-Fordism may involve mass production, mass consumption and mass welfare – but organised in an integrated manner rather than involving separate employment and contract rights for separate 'guilds' or cadres of workers and professionals which characterised the heavily unionised economy of the 1970s). Thus in the NHS we see employment and labour force initiatives such as 'Agenda for Change' which represent standardisation rather than local flexibility.

An overwhelming reason for the decline of Keynesian National Welfare State (as agreed by both the New Right and the Marxisant Left) was a falling rate of profit in the economy accompanied by inflation which led to a vicious circle in terms of wage demands and legitimacy. Applying national pay norms and conditions across whole industrial sectors which couldn't necessarily afford them was a feature of the old 'regime' which yielded to the post-Fordist economy and flexibility.

The choice had been to reinvigorate capitalism or make a transition to socialism. The latter was never likely. The only political mechanism for effecting it was the Labour Party. While the 'alternative economic strategy' as a left social democratic variant of capitalism had intellectual power (Eatwell, 1982), by the time it was bolted on to the 'left programme' of the Bennites in the Labour Party, it was wholly implausible and unrealistic (Radice, 2002, pp 262-3), and led in the end to 'the longest suicide note in history' (the 1983 Labour Party Manifesto).

The paradox for an institution such as the NHS is that it must be both Fordist and post-Fordist: as Derek Wanless, Gordon Brown's chosen health advisor, has put it, the NHS admittedly cannot provide a five star service, but must produce at least a three star standard (standardised?) service for everyone if it is to meet expectations while also be affordable. The implications for the labour force are neo-Fordist rather than post-Fordist. At the same time, if the NHS is to fulfil its economic as well as its social mission (and also fulfil its 'consumerist' mission for the better off), it must provide differentiated services according to differentiated needs and demands in a more inegalitarian society.

Political Economy, Healthcare and The State

It is not far-fetched to draw a comparison between the political economy of Labour in the late 1920s and early 1930s and Tony Blair's New Labour. Then as now, Labour was obsessed, under Prime Minister McDonald, with appearing fiscally responsible, and was also in hock to the macro- economic orthodoxy of the day. Then it was pre-Keynesian supply-side economics; today it is post-Keynesian supply-side economics. The Third Way, as an economic strategy at least, has proved ephemeral.

Of course the world economy operated differently in some ways. Britain was losing its place as a primary exporter, early in the century; today, Britain has to fight for its share of inward investment. But the meaning is the same for British workers – intensified labour, or unemployment. It might be thought New Labour has an answer to this – education and skills training, to put us at the elite end of today's globalised world economy. But this is as partial a solution as Chancellor Snowden's 'support for export industries' as the answer in 1929. As that unorthodox modern buccaneer James Goldsmith put it (1994), skilled labour in the developing world can still outbid our own labour. Britain gets rich today by 'British' and multi-national companies transferring production abroad – that is, national wealth is defined as profit for capital. And it can get worse than that: as fairly-paid labour is eliminated, demand falls; companies fold; and only the hyper-rich corporations prosper.

For the poor countries of the world ('developing' is a euphemism), globalisation is bringing problems as well as opportunities – and even the latter have a sting in the tail. Some of the problems are of course caused by hypocrisy in parts of the developed world: the rhetoric of open markets is belied by the reality of dumping subsidised goods in poor countries. And markets for primary products from the developing world need to be opened more.

But some problems are intrinsic to capitalist globalisation: elites in poor countries seek to import more expensive but more cost-effective goods from the developed world; in turn, elite industries in poor countries are geared to the export market; and there are shrinking national and local economies from which the poor can benefit as producers and consumers. Add to this the expropriation of natural resources through patenting and other devices under the tutelage of the World Trade Organisation, and we realise that, to benefit the poor, globalisation would have to be transformed.

The political constituency for this has to come from the 'losers' in rich countries making common cause with the losers in poor countries. The trouble is that political strategy in the rich countries makes these losers a minority of the voting classes. This can even be true in poor countries, where globalisation can make a critical mass of people 'better-off' but more intensively exploited. Any 'answer' requires global trade rules to be challenged such that industry in the developed world is legitimately protected while markets are opened to legitimately-produced goods from the developing world. This is logically possible but politically very difficult, when the politics of international relations and trade are accounted for – making recent UN shenanigans over Iraq simple by comparison!

Yet if we take material needs (housing; food; education; health; clean environment; work/life balance and related community stability) as the touchstone, many workers and families are actually getting poorer. It is only when we add an obsolete-as-soon-as-it's-invented technology that 'the standard of living is rising for all but the bottom ten per cent' in the West.

Post-Fordism and Public Policy

What was called post-Fordism in the early 1990s was basically the class (economic and social) structures deriving within nations from increasingly international capitalist political economy and the 'regulation' strategies of governments to compete in open markets. This led to literature in political science (state theory) on the alleged 'hollowing out' of the state, now christened the 'Schumpeterian workfare state' (Jessop, 2002) and to the new orthodoxy in public administration of 'governance' (emphasis on the gerundive). The latter reflected a world in which direct government, provision, administration and/or management by the state had allegedly been replaced by a more softly-softly role for the state in steering and regulating a more fragmented, pluralised, privatised and/or non-hierarchical polity.

Whatever the link between the changing 'regime' in political economy, based on the so-called regulation theory of Aglietta (1979; 1982) and others and the changing policy functions of the state, a particular question arose as to the nature of the welfare state – in a nutshell, was it post-Fordist also?

The main thesis is that economic globalisation has significant, if sometimes uneven, effects. Global capitalism is the main influence upon national economies in today's world, and political economy is the most significant determinant of health policy in a number of significant senses.

Firstly, it heavily influences how much money is available for public healthcare systems and how such revenue is raised (from whom) i.e. the prospects for equitably-funded and adequately-financed health services.

Secondly, it influences who benefits most from publicly funded services: are they available to everybody on the basis of clinical and social needs (i.e. the social or ethical mission) or is access influenced by economic considerations (such as the need for a healthy workforce, or the need to invest in particular cadres of employees)?

Thirdly, globalisation adds a layer onto the so-called post-Fordist economic and social structure, whereby mass production and mass welfare has been replaced by a differentiated economy and society with greater income inequality. In this context, health services must compete with the rest of the economy for skilled labour. This often creates budgetary problems for public health services, as will be discussed below.

The implications of these trends are explored for a variety of types of healthcare system in a variety of types of economy. The division of the world into 'developed' and 'developing' countries is inappropriate, as is the outdated categorisation into first, second and third worlds. Global capitalism means (to resurrect a phrase) combined and uneven development, in which so-called developed countries have 'Third World'-style **laagers** – as in the USA – and so-called developing countries (like Brazil) have highly advanced niches in their economies. In other words, the national economy and nation state have both less autonomy and less homogeneity in today's world. This chapter elucidates the implications of such trends for healthcare systems.

The Political Economy of Global Capitalism

The thirty 'boom years' from 1945 to 1975 in (what were then called) Western countries were the archetypal years of the industrial welfare state. Economically and fiscally, mass production, mass consumption and mass welfare were the order of the day. Politically, it was the heyday of social democracy. As regards the rest of the world, of course, it was a different story: the West's social democracy depended economically upon cheap primary products (and in particular cheap oil) from developing countries. Yet it was also the time of 'three worlds' – the First World of the superpowers; the Second World of Europe, West and East; and the Third World, the (allegedly) developing world.

'Post-Fordist capitalism' is in fact the part-economic, part-political, part-technological phenomenon which has characterised the development of 'advanced capitalism' in the years since the long boom. Post-Fordism refers to the decline of mass manufacturing (and the industrial welfare state to which it gave birth as a result of the predominance of the working class in the electorate at that time). The economy and society are more differentiated; and a combination of technological development and the dynamics of capitalism have seen both the export of 'industrial production' on the one hand, and the hybrid society of specialised niche production and unskilled laagers, in countries like the UK, on the other hand.

For our purposes, in exploring the effects upon welfare and in particular health policy, the political consequences of post-Fordism (and that is not to take any particular viewpoint as to its causes or detailed characteristics) are: the decline of the 'left-wing majority' based on the manufacturing working class being a majority within the voting public; and, the rise of the contented majority' as characterised by the voting publics which produced the Thatcher governments in the UK and the Reagan Presidencies in the United States. The contented majority is a phrase coined by John Kenneth Galbraith (*op, cit*) to refer to the fact that, of those who vote a majority now have an economic stake in the status quo (or perceived themselves to have). In the somewhat discredited sequential language of 'first, second and third ways', the first way was the industrial welfare state, the second way was Thatcherism (in a UK context) – and the question remains as to whether there is a third way or what it might be.

My argument is that, as global capitalism continues its excavations of economy and cultures, the era of the contented majority has given way to the era of the insecure majority. To put it bluntly, people cannot see a way out of global capitalism (whether they wish to or not), but are disquieted consciously or otherwise by a variety of its manifestations. Employment is less secure even when it is better paid; exploitation is intensified, even when incomes are higher; and – crucial for the current essay – more 'welfare state' (in particular health and education) is sought by a majority yet the means of mobilising the revenue to achieve that is problematical.

In a nutshell, if people – 'swing voter' strata – wanted to trade a bit of income for security, it is unlikely that they would see the political or economic route to so doing. That is why, in the UK, 'New Labour is New Labour' irrespective of the values of its proponents (clearly Blair welcomes such trends; more socialist-minded Labour politicians such as the Cooks, Becketts and Shorts of this world presumably less so).

The Political Economy of Healthcare

The issue for healthcare systems is actually three-fold as discussed above. Let us now analyse these points more. The **first** consideration is the generation of revenue for public healthcare systems. A publicly funded National Health Service as in the UK or Sweden, funded from taxation, requires an adequately-progressive tax system to generate enough revenue to provide a generously-provided health service adequate to the needs of a majority of citizens. The middle classes will only get what they want from the health service if it is well enough funded to minimise waiting lists and waiting times (same for the poorer elements of society; it is just that they have no alternative in terms of recourse to the private sector). Yet taxes will only be progressive if politics permits (see below).

A progressive tax system may threaten a country's position within global capitalism: higher taxes may discourage inward investment and hasten the export of capital. If taxes were placed directly on the corporate sector, clearly this is likely, in a Dutch auction for inward investment and the retention of existing investment. If taxes were placed on personal income, then they will clearly be resisted by the better off: the question is whether the better off can form a majority political/electoral coalition as in the era of the contented majority. Even if they cannot, the middle and lower ranks of earners may also resist higher taxes on the grounds that – whether they are working a lot harder for a little more money, or actually receiving less money in real terms – lower taxes are a means of compensating for such a situation. One has the additional consideration that poorer tax payers are less willing to pay tax the less progressive the system is i.e. proportionate have to pay more.

To mobilise either a progressive tax system or a tax system which generates enough money to provide (let us say in the UK context) a National Health Service funded generously enough to prevent the adverse comparisons in terms of spending with say Germany and France, is therefore no easy business. Even when the 'contented majority' is not dominant, firstly, a majority of voters may see 'no alternative' to the low tax, national economy competing in a global environment; and, secondly, even if alternatives are perceived, then disengaging from such a global environment may be seen as an untenable national protectionism (the 'alternative economic strategy' is long buried) or alternatively dependent upon the maintenance of regional blocks such as the European Union. The latter, in turn, would, however, have to take a much clearer stance as to how they would reconcile its 'social model' or the modern welfare state with the political economy of the world. All in all, it is easy to see why fatalism persists in politics and why underfunding of public services is the key issue of the age for social democrats.

The **second** consideration is access to services. Within the time of constrained public National Health Service, for example, access to services may be simply on the basis of clinical needs – but with 'rationing' and long waiting times – or on the basis of criteria other than simply clinical need (whether these criteria are admitted by politicians, and others, or not). For example: competition in the post-Fordist globalised capitalist economy may benefit from selective state investment in enterprise.

That is, global capitalism is not simply the era of the minimal state – but neither is it the era of the state operating on universal principles. It is the era of the 'competition state' or the pragmatic, opportunist state. There is a perfectly plausible neo-Marxist argument which would argue that the state and global capitalism is likely to invest in 'cheap health services', based on extracting surplus value from health workers, to provide infrastructure (i.e. healthy workers) which increase both the profitability of enterprise and the attractiveness of the country as a location of enterprise as a result. This could even sound progressive – invest in your workers and your country will be more competitive.

The sting in the tale is that the investment, if carried out rationally, will not be universal: it will be a case of investing in particular cadres of workers, or in particular sectors of the economy where there are shortages of skilled workers and so on and so forth. In other words, selective state investment does via the public sector what the American healthcare system does privately: firms invest in their workers, including in the healthcare of these workers, where it is necessary to do so; and not where it is not. Good quality health insurance is both an investment in and a perk for i.e. a recruitment tool), for skilled and scarce workers and managers in the United States. Cheap labour doesn't get health insurance – it is easier to replace such workers than to invest in them. The argument that the mobility of scarce/skilled workers would discourage investment is diminished when one considers that such investment also provides a perk – it is actually an attempt to 'lock in' such workers to the company, and so forth.

If, in a country like the UK, the state invests in workers via the public sector, the implication for the NHS – whatever the rhetoric – the less skilled, the less useful, the old and so forth will receive less investment. Note that there is no claim by the author that this is happening in a systematic manner – but it may be 'emergent strategy' … and it may even be the internal logic of what sounds much more progressive when described by Anthony Giddens (1998) as the 'third way'.

Thirdly, one must consider employment. Public health services will have to compete to attract workers. From the very beginning of the chain, medical students and other potential professionals will choose their education according to alternative options, in turn linked to alternative economic possibilities to some extent. Salaries and conditions in the health service will condition the health service's ability to compete within the economy generally, both national and international. At the end of the day, the limited public service budget can pay enough to train and recruit the skilled/scarce workers (e.g. doctors in particular specialties) or pay living wages to the poorer unskilled workers, or see limits placed upon numbers in each category as a result of failing way structures out of the economy as a whole. That in a nutshell is what the NHS sees with its various staff shortages, over time ranging from one discipline to another – depending upon the political priorities of the day (rather like punching the balloon in terms of the problem reappearing within another cadre of worker).

Putting the three considerations together (the political economy of financing public health services; priorities in access to services; and employment considerations), we can see that keeping the better off 'on board' the NHS means providing a comprehensive National Health Service which provides quality treatment in a timely manner. And for the worse off – those whose labour is expendable – there is a requirement to provide rescue and care through the National Health Service, if it is to be a humanitarian social institution and not just a desiccated calculating machine. Paradoxically therefore, economists' panaceas such as 'cost utility analysis' to decide who gets healthcare and who doesn't, are pretty unhelpful as regards the political project for the NHS, considering the viewpoint of both middle classes and the poor. Both have to get ready access without technocratically-decided denials of care, or the political constituency for the NHS is undermined. Healthcare is an exceptional service with exceptional (yet justified) expectations.

Britain versus Europe?

It is a paradox that, even as the UK was agonising about whether the NHS is or ought to be sustainable for the 21st Century, continental systems such as those in France – which enjoy lots of domestic popularity – were adapting some of the planning mechanisms of Beveridge systems such as the National Health Service. These mechanisms include regional planning agencies for hospital care (both public and private); the pooling of insurance funds to ensure more global purchasing; and so on. Clearly the level of financing is crucial. France spends 11% of its GDP on health compared to Britain's 7% (rising). When one looks at the source of France's social insurance, one finds significant payment by employers as well as individuals towards the statutory system. Even though there is more 'private top-up' than in Britain, the statutory public system still spends substantially more than does the NHS.

Paradoxically again, a move towards to a national health service in a country like France could actually mean less progressive means of funding the system: the less progressive income tax is, the less progressive is the National Health Service option (in terms of redistributing from rich to poor) as compared to (for example) France's system of significant employer contributions to social and health insurance. In other words, a National Health Service (the Beveridge model (Paton et al, 2000)) can actually be favoured by business and perhaps government as a means of lessening the burden on industry. The question that arises, of course, in the case of a country like France is, does a generous social wage (payment into statutory schemes by employers, for example) mean less generous incomes. Free market economists in the United States have often made the argument that statutory health insurance in the United States would simply mean lower wages as the money was contributed by employers in other ways. Further research on this question is needed in Europe.

The present author believes that the NHS could spend half the difference between its level of health spending and the levels in France and Germany and – as a result of the intrinsic efficiency and effectiveness of NHS style spending – achieve as good results as these countries. The danger is that, with an inadequate service, better off voters will only support these elements of the NHS which they feel they can secure more cheaply as well as promptly through the public service. That is, the NHS will be eroded towards a core – and perhaps emergency service in the long run if we do not 'get the political economy right'.

New Labour's increasingly desperate attempts, after their big election victory of 2001, to make the NHS more palatable to better off citizens suggests that history is repeating itself: Mrs Thatcher had just been handsomely re-elected in 1987 when the crisis that led to her review of the National Health Service was perceived to have begun. Today's crisis consists in the need to provide both prompt and high quality treatment. Hence ideas about patients allegedly being allowed to 'go anywhere' for care, including abroad.

Some commentators have depicted those ideas as reinvigoration of Thatcher's internal market, although that is not the case – in its aspirations, the policy is more about free movement of patients with the money being found to pay for their care. The Thatcher internal market was in fact about restrictions upon mobility, in line with contracts with purchasers and providers. Indeed one could argue that Labour's blind alley has been due to the extent to which it has partially continued the Thatcher reforms. Presumably it was in this vein that the then French Health Minister Bernard Kouchner criticised Tony Blair and then-Health Secretary Alan Milburn vigorously in *The New Statesman* in September 2001 (September 21st) on the grounds that what the NHS needed was more money and less privatisation.

Interestingly Kouchner depicted his own system as a public system, without the 'privatisation' trappings such as the Private Finance Initiative and the like that we see in Britain. Yet in Britain, the French system is seen as an example of 'greater private involvement'. There is frequent misunderstanding in the UK as to the structure and dynamics of the French system – which is intrinsically public in terms of financing, and also public in terms of regulatory control of the pre-existing private sector. Britain's privatisation initiatives are taking the NHS in an altogether different direction, (and, in the view of this author, in a half-baked manner).

Chapter 2

The State, Post Fordism and Health Services

The State

The very phrase 'theory of the state' has a 1970s feel to it. It conjures up *inter alia* the ghosts of debates within Marxism about matters such as the relative autonomy of the state, and the role of the state in capitalist society. Some such state theory was overly 'metaphysical' and arguably unfalsifiable (e.g. Poulantzas, 1973). Yet debates about the theory of the state, at their best, were useful in illuminating how power in policy and implementation was related to economic power: the power of capital was always more fundamental than mainstream Anglo-American political science allowed.

By the new millennium, global capitalism has replaced (national) 'capitalist society' as the focus of attention for those seeking to explain the behaviour of 'the state' and the nature of public policy. This time, there is less of a rarefied debate characterised by over-theoretical 'isms', the absence of which no doubt reflecting what might be termed the 'new end of ideology.' Marxisant approaches such as 'regulation theory' and the concepts of the 'Schumpeterian workfare state' and the 'competition state' (Cerny and Evans, 1998) are arguably little more than a re-description of changing capitalism, as opposed to deeper explanation, but are nevertheless useful in focusing the mind upon the constraints facing domestic economic policy and the welfare state (Coates and Hay, 2000) Meanwhile, in the political mainstream, there is a gulf between the rhetoric of the 'Third Way' and those very constraints upon policy in today's global capitalist world. To put it another way, proponents of the third way signal left and turn right when they come to the international traffic-lights.

It is therefore worth re-examining the state's role in policy. We are in a 'third phase' of post-war capitalism which leads to major difficulties for the continuing viability of equitable public health services. In Britain, the health service is at the core of the welfare state. If the NHS's role is changed over time, then we can reasonably assume that the rest of the welfare state is even more malleable in the interests of 'the economy' i.e. survivability in a global capitalist world or whatever. What is the state's role in this?

Despite the different healthcare systems across the world, the role of the state in healthcare is increasingly construed as promoting competitiveness in the capitalist world economy. While countries clearly differ as their social objectives and as to the prevailing degree of equity in access to healthcare, the trend is to a set of 'minimum services' in healthcare for either the poor or the general population, on the one hand, and wider access to better services as investment in core workers and consumption by the better-off, on the other hand. The state is increasing its role in the former and diminishing its role in the latter. To present the former as evidence of increasing equity is therefore misleading.

Countries such as the UK and Sweden are 'bucking the trend' to the extent that they maintain genuinely universal and comprehensive public health services (as opposed to skewing the priorities within their socialised systems to maintain the allegiance of the better-off). It is thus an open question as to how sustainable such systems are in the environment of laisser-faire global capitalism. This was the broad context within which the British 'internal market' in the NHS was developed, sometimes referred to as a 'quasi-market.' (Bartlett and le Grand, Eds., 1993)

The state's role in healthcare financing and provision and in the promotion of health was seen as a growing one in the twentieth century, until the last twenty years. Not only was the protection of the poor and uninsured a central plank of social democracy but the rising cost of increasingly complex medical care in the twentieth century meant that even the well-off benefited from public insurance or financing. Only recently has the post-war orthodoxy of an expanding public healthcare state (Moran, 1999) been overturned, as globalisation (here meaning global capitalism) has changed the political economy and public policy of nation-states. In the West, if we can still use that term, the industrial welfare state has yielded to 'post-Fordism' and the 'competition state'. The state now has a facilitating role in securing employment for its citizens (sector by sector; niche by niche) rather than planning the terms and conditions of that employment. In the rest of the world, including the former Eastern block, state-financed health services are under pressure, as capitalism, prevailing ideology and health sector reform diminish the prospects for collectivism.

Three Phases of Capitalism

To expand the above discussion, what might be termed the 'first phase' of post-war capitalism in Western Europe was the era of the industrial welfare state, as introduced above. The working class was more homogeneous, based largely upon national industrial manufacturing. There was a political capacity for redistributive social policy, as a 'left-of-centre' electoral majority prevailed (even under the stewardship of Conservative or right-of-centre parties). The economic capacity for redistribution was however limited over time, as analysed in the 'fiscal crisis' literature of both right and left: capitalism required adequate profit (Bacon and Eltis, 1976) and social investment vied with social expenses (O'Connor, 1973) or 'legitimation.' More optimistically, it could be argued that this 'first phase' redistributed enough if the 'social contract' between labour and capital operated as in Sweden. But this was before modern globalisation.

The second phase was the era of the contented majority (Galbraith, *op. cit*) when the electoral majority was right-of-centre. This was the era of Thatcherism-Reaganism in the West and the 'World Bank rampant' in the Rest. In the political economy of Thatcherism, the actual beneficiaries of revived capitalism were joined politically by the temporary beneficiaries, the economically aspirant and the ideologically-converted. There was the economic capacity to redistribute, but not the political (electoral) capacity. This was the era when the UK became a market leader in 'health sector reform' applied to government health services. Again, more optimistically, it could be argued that the 'second phase' only required limited redistribution to the 'losers' without severe loss of income by the gains. This was the basis – in the UK – for the New Labour agenda.

The third phase is the contemporary phase where greater globally-induced economic insecurity can lead either to right or left coalitions, depending upon whether maintenance of position or security is sought. If the pivotal social and voting strata 'swing left' there may be a domestic political capacity for a redistributive policy. Yet the economic capacity for such action at the nation-state level or lower will be constrained by globalisation. The Labour victory in the UK in 1997, for example, probably reflected the desire to 'have one's cake and eat it' on the part of previously Conservative-voting strata i.e. a desire for greater economic security and a 'kindler and gentler' Britain (to follow Labour Cabinet Minister David Blunkett in quoting George Bush Sr.) while seeking to retain of the fruits of Thatcherism. Yet the compatibility of global capitalism with the security of 'one nation' is in doubt.

Global Capitalism and Health Sector Reform

Countries attract inward investment and prevent outflows of capital by running economies based on lower wages or intensified labour (higher productivity) or both. Lower wages mean lower taxes for workers to seek to preserve their take-home pay; higher productivity means fewer workers and less tax-yield. Either way, there is less of a tax base for expanding public expenditure, unless 'swing' voters overtly choose slightly lower income in turn for greater security and (perhaps) more leisure. More rapidly, if the downward pressure on wages is halted by the taming of globalisation, then taxation becomes less of a burden.

The 'logic' of globalisation has been transmitted directly to the world of health policy. For example, a 'think tank' of leading businessmen from multi-national corporations in Europe in the mid-1980s, setting out just this rationale (Warner, in Lee (Ed.), 1994), had as one of its members a certain Dekker, from the Phillips group in the Netherlands, who also chaired the Dutch health reform committee leading to the Dekker plan of 1987 (which was partially implemented over the 1990s albeit in a restricted form). The Dutch model of 'managed competition' became the prototype for reform of Bismarckian social insurance schemes – in Europe and beyond (e.g.

South America) as well as for the failed Clinton Plan in the US (Paton, 1996). The UK model of internal markets and purchaser/provider splits in tax-funded Beveridge or government health systems was devised by right-wing advisers and politicians who advocated commercialisation in the public sector.

The assumption was that publicly-funded healthcare had to be delivered more efficiently, or cheaply, and had to be more carefully targeted. In Western countries such as the Netherlands, the latter could be done by advocating publicly-funded universal access for a restricted basket of services (i.e. universality but not comprehensiveness). In the 'developing' world from the 1980s onwards, usually under the aegis of multi-lateral agencies such as the World Bank and bi-lateral aid departments such as Britain's Overseas Development Administration (which became the Department for International Development in 1997), 'Western' policies promoting market forces in healthcare have been advocated and partially implemented. In other developing countries, the watchword has been 'decentralisation', but the political intention has frequently been both to limit the role of the state in healthcare and to make communities more responsible for their own health (which sounds culturally progressive but is likely to be fiscally regressive.)

A general consequence of global capitalism – and national capitalist regimes using global capitalism as an excuse for increased inequality – is that lower wages and intensified labour are not compensated by lower prices (Paton, 2000). It might seem to be a paradox that firms can still be fighting to survive after lowering wages, intensifying their workers' labour and 'reprofiling' their workforces both to 'upskill' and 'deskill' where appropriate. Here however we must make a distinction between multi-national companies and 'stock exchange' companies, on the one hand, and wholly-owned national firms , on the other hand. In the former sector, ever-higher profits are needed, otherwise investment dries up: it is a case of 'up or out.' Lower wages do not lead to lower prices, as a generalisation – that is not what is driving the need for lower wages; instead a greater exploitation of labour is needed to achieve higher profit. In the latter sector, investment is harder to come by, as the Anglo-American model of capitalism drives out alternative models in the era of globalisation. The German model et al are crowded out. This happens both as the behaviour of banks and economic institutions changes and as a result of the 'competitive single market policies' of organisations such as the European Union and the World Trade Organisation.

Social Investment or Post-Fordist Capitalism?

Shorn of its more pretentious or banal rhetoric, the 'third way' has been presented in the UK as a means of avoiding traditional 'tax and spend' social democracy without (re)lapsing into Thatcherism. Social democracy, never mind socialism, is caricatured as contrasting the dictates of the economy and social equity, and favouring the latter to the disadvantage of the former. The 'third way' however is alleged to treat the two together in a common purpose. It implies that social equity is compatible with globalisation. Giddens for example (1998) has talked of the 'social investment state.' In the health arena, the implication is that the state has a role in promoting health in ways which help the economy.

In this sense, there is little new; indeed such a claim is either banal or pre-dated by twentieth-century Marxist views of welfare. There is a familiar distinction between healthcare as investment and as consumption, as well as between either or both of these on an individual, class or social basis. The Marxist view of the British National Health Service, for example, can see it as tending to state subsidy of capital, and cheap investment in a healthy workforce, even if it was created in socialist struggle (Navarro, 1978). The Marxist view of welfare distinguished between social capital and social expenses, with a tendency to fiscal crisis occasioned by the inability of the state to do both while also letting private capital prosper (O'Connor, 1973). Marx distinguished between productive and unproductive labour in terms of whether it created capital (through surplus value) or spent capital (as with marketing.) Today however this distinction is less useful (Braverman, 1974) and the NHS is a good example : it is paid *inter alia* from taxes of profits but it creates increased profit as a service to the health of workers to which these workers' employers pay less than they benefit.

The question can then arise, of course : if the NHS model is useful for capitalism, why does it not find its apotheosis in the home of capitalism, the USA? The answer, on Marxist terms, would have to be that, especially in the historical absence of socialist struggle, there are other means of investing in the workforce which capital(ists) may prefer for other reasons. For example, in the USA, an NHS would mean paying for many who are currently uninsured. Firms may use healthcare benefits as perks or recruitment incentives for favoured workers (Greer, 1998) as a well as a means on investing in their own workforce; and cheap and plentiful workers are replaceable and so investment in their health is not necessary. Firms may not follow their 'rational' economic self-interest (getting the state to pay for healthcare by taxing others more) for ideological reasons (belief in the market and self-sufficiency).

Crucially, both health corporations and individual health 'entrepreneurs' in the US are, a representative part of mainstream capitalism and an important political constituency. The U.S.'s 'capitalist state' is structured such that direct influence by capitalist constituencies is more significant than in the UK. This means that the predominance of financing (and therefore cost – control) which we see in the UK is less in the U.S. The 'provision' lobby is powerful in aggregate (whether HMOs or defenders of fee service medicine). In the UK where most provision is within the NHS, the 'provision lobby' is within the NHS and is in effect part of the state, or rather an irritant fly on the back of the state elephant. It has no independent power, except a limited power to shape 'managerialist' policy by influencing Ministers if the latter are so inclined.

Overall, health sector reform in the US has been business-driven, with 'managed care' both an attempt by general business to control costs and a consequence of the search for monopoly in the healthcare industry (both payers and providers, and networks of both). But it is at least arguable that general business (although clearly not the healthcare industry) would benefit from publicly-owned health services from which the state extracted a 'surplus value' on behalf of general business.

In other words, there is nothing new – or **necessarily** progressive – about using the state to invest in health. It is argued here that the 'third way' – a role for the state but without generalised 'tax and spend' – is in fact the direct descendant of the approach which the rational capitalist state would follow according to 1970s-style Marxist analysis. It is simply that the means of investing in the workforce, on behalf of industry, varies as the structure of the workforce changes. The 'third way' is the political post-hoc rationalisation of what the capitalist state must do. That is why there is inevitable tension between its origin and the aspirations of its more idealistic proponents who seek to incorporate more radical policy prescriptions within it – with Anthony Giddens (1998) straddling the divide, as it were!

Moreover the conceptualisation of 'civil society' made in the 'third way' is a limited one, and arguably an illiberal one. The collective or communitarian action which is the 'third way' between individualism and statism is action 'in the private realm' i.e. beyond the state and (in this case) outside the workplace. Yet political liberalism is based on a 'private realm' within which men are free to act (subject to not harming others). There are constraints on the origansation of work, either agreed in an explicit or implicit 'social contract' which sets out principles of economic or social organisation or – more likely – because all men are not equally free to determine their employment and life-chances. But outside this realm, political and cultural freedom exists.

The third way philosophy however, like the communitarian philosophy on which it draws, prescribes how time is to be spent in that private realm – indeed the approach has been whimsically summed up by le Grand (1998) as 'CORA' (to mimic Mrs. Thatcher's TINA – There Is No Alternative), which stands for Community, Opportunity, Responsibility and Authority. The price of limited opportunity, one might say, is acceptance not just of community authority (prescribed, moreover, from on high) but of the responsibility to organize 'voluntarily' to build social capital. Yet the better-off don't rely on policy to 'create' social capital – they don't need it (or sometimes they have it automatically).

The costs of collective and communitarian organization are relatively higher for the poor : lower incomes and more pressure on time means that the 'opportunity cost' of activism is high; and expecting the poor to solve their own problems is fiscally regressive. As a result benefits would need to very high, or rather immediately tangible, for such activism to be undertaken let alone sustained. 'Pilot projects' and 'special schemes' are therefore likely to wither on the vine unless converted into permanent, general programmes. But it was the desire to avoid such 'tax and spend' which led to the 'piecemeal' approach in the first place, despite evidence from the US that the 'radical' yet piecemeal programmes of the 'Great Society' in the 1960s had very limited success (the partial exceptions being those which applied to all e.g. Headstart). Although often sneered-at at a central policy level by left-wing intellectuals, 'third way' initiatives today may even attract a little 'radical chic' on the ground (although not as much as in the 1960s): social activists, if they can't get the programmes they love, tend to love the programmes they've got, and 'spin' accordingly. Yet radical chic may end up pretty conservative.

The third way moreover presents a very bourgeois picture of civil society. Capitalism exists : that's a given. The nature of work is not a matter of social choice: that's a given. Therefore community action is in a strictly limited sphere. What is more, the need to extract the maximum value (and surplus value) out of public services leads to increasing inspectorate and central control, as the only possible alternative to 'internal markets' and the like which are either expensive or merely a smokescreen for central control. (Paton et al, 1998) This leaves the 'third way' as more 'command and control' than the first way ever was – and indeed ensures that the broader economic 'third way' (or rather, the capitalist state run by a Labour government) squeezes out the NHS-specific 'third way' (i.e. collaboration rather than either the market or 'command and control', which was always a topsy-turvy characterisation of the evolving history of the NHS).

The New End of Ideology

The 'end of ideology' in the 1960s and early 1970s (Bell, 1960) referred to the alleged convergence of Western capitalism (the first way) and Eastern communism (the second way) through the pluralization of the latter and the 'social democratisation' of the former – accompanied by a fleeting 'detente'. This was the original third way. The subsequent events of the 1980s and 1990s show how transitory the conventional wisdoms of both sociology and political science can be. Today we have a 'new end of ideology', which the likes of Clinton, Blair and Schröder liked at least temporarily to call the third way or the neue mitte. But whereas the earlier one was based upon political convergence and political choice, today's is based upon the seeming inevitability of global capitalism : 'there is no alternative'. The earlier 'social trends' were in part based on political autonomy; today's are based on its abrogation. The earlier 'third way' was social democracy, after (first) Victorian capitalism and (secondly) communism.

Today's third way is inverted – it follows (first) social democratic planning and (second) Thatcherism; and attempts to combine the economics of the latter with (some of) the social aspirations of the former.

The Changing Capitalist State and Healthcare Reform ...

To recap: paradoxically, the **capacity** of the 'healthcare state' (Moran, 1999) is increasing in proportion to the complexity of social regulation, while the state's **autonomy** from economic interests is diminishing. Either the 'new 'managerialism' (Exworthy and Halford (eds), 1999) or direct politicisation of public sector targets is used is to seek to tailor health services to both economic needs and economically-determined social needs. It is argued here that use of the central state to extract maximum additional 'surplus value' for private business from healthcare provision reaches its apotheosis in the NHS model. Two paradoxes therefore arise. Firstly, the most progressive and egalitarian model for health services (the NHS model) is also the most easily subverted. (The central state can be used and abused). Secondly, where the NHS model is 'off the political agenda', surrogate policy for 'taming healthcare' in the interests of business is much less effective. This latter situation pertains in the 'Bismarckian', or social insurance, systems of Europe.

'Regulation Theory', Post-Fordism, And The NHS

Regarding 'regulation (regime) theory' (Aglietta, *op. cit*), and the more specific postulate of post-Fordism (Jessop, *op. cit*), the case of national health services (illustrated by the British NHS) suggests that the concept of the 'post-Fordist welfare state may be somewhat wide of the mark.

Changing political economy there has undoubtedly been. The industrial welfare state has yielded to the differentiated political economy, in 'advanced Western' countries, characterised by Stages 2 and 3 in Part 2 above. This is related to changing relationships and patterns of production and consumption in the world economy rather than to some intrinsic move to post-industrial society or some 'gee whiz' facet of the so-called knowledge economy (if there be such, its organisation can be politically contested).

But the most effective means for health services to be organised 'for' this economy (and the question is begged: is this a functionalist view or an instrumentalist/power-analytical view? – see below) may well be in a 'Fordist' or 'neo-Fordist' manner. If post-Fordism means simply more private consumption and therefore new 'products' in health care, produced under new 'relations of production', it is both a pretentious re-writing of the obvious and also banal. The key question is what happens to health services in the public sector, e.g. in the English NHS, or in the quasi-public sector, in countries such as France and Germany i.e. in countries where publicly-financed services predominate.

Using the concepts of regulation theory (synthesizing Jessop's (1994(a); 1994(b); 1999; 2002) different writings in applying such), are such services: (1) mass produced and/or (2) flexibly produced? (3) Does a new regime of accumulation mean new relations of production e.g. a move from Keynesian full employment to selective investment in economic niches)? And if there is such a move economy-wide, is it replicated in the NHS? For example, do new 'workforce initiatives' such as Agenda for Change seek both to increase integration and control of the workforce (Braverman, 2000) **and** to change power relations (see below). Since the NHS is a 'support service' to the capitalist economy rather than a locus for core capital-labour relations, changing relations may be relative rather than fundamental: that is, we may see diminished power for organised labour and increased power for other cadres, but varying contingently. (4) Is there a transition from the national to the international in terms of the state's focus and therefore its role? (5) Are the power relations, or compromise, between capital and labour changed? (6) Is there a move from state policy and its implementation to regime governance? (7) What are the social and political 'means of enforcement' of the new regime, if there be one?

In fact the NHS in England is moving (firstly) from pre-Fordism to Fordism, in some respects; and (secondly) from classical Fordism to neo-Fordism, in others. Firstly, doctors have been – and sometimes still are – organised in guilds, under the umbrella of the NHS. Recent reforms have sought to manage their performance in line with 'output' objectives and to create – through 'collaborative' mechanisms – their integration into the wider workforce. But these reforms are still at the aspirational level.

Secondly, other professions and 'non-professional workers' have resembled, in the past, in widely varying degrees, the 'Fordist' model more closely, in that they have been subject both to the expectations (of the state and managers) and to control. Admittedly there has been a difference between the industrial model of 'Fordism' and the health (and perhaps general welfare) model: the former has tended to involve integrated production even where workforces were differentiated internally; and the latter has involved only partial 'Fordism' in that each profession or cadre has been managed separately. Yet even in private (especially manufacturing) industry, different cadres based on crafts and skills often organised themselves (especially via trade unions during the heyday of social democracy) for 'producer' purposes rather than 'consumer' interests. To that extent, there is a parallel with the 'welfare industry'.

In both sectors, now, a key change is from the 'autonomy' of labour to the 'necessities' of both competition and the need for super-profits in (especially) the international business sector. Whether this means 'post Fordism' (the end of mass production *et al*) or 'neo Fordism' (increased surplus value from mass production though new means of organisation of labour, especially the interaction at different cadres) is a moot point.

Regarding the tenets of regulation theory (above, (1) to (7)):

(1) the trend in the NHS has been to an integration of mass production. We have gone from the 'pre-Fordism' of guilds in the healthcare production process to the 'neo-Fordism' of a more corporately-integrated production process, or rather the beginnings of such. Confusingly this is happening in the post-Fordist era as regards the wider economy.

(2) Flexible production, in some cases flexible specialisation, is sometimes but not always a countervailing trend – health services have always been differentiated products (whether or not for differentiated consumers), and now the trend is to produce the services more 'scientifically.' This may lead to more 'mass production' or to differentiated production processes and rewards under 'flexible specialisation'. In the NHS, 'choice' tends to consist in mechanistic choice between homogenised 'products' with differentiated 'frills' (if that) – managed (i.e. restricted) by 'commissioning' agents of the state. (Any student

of the NHS's 'Choose and Book' initiative of 2006 will get the picture!)

(3) Regarding the new regime of accumulation, this operates at the level of the macro-economy. The implication for welfare/health, in the public sector, is that of 'doing more for less', rather than necessarily a new dynamic within the welfare/health sector to mirror the economy-wide dynamic. Whether more is achieved for less through Fordism, neo-Fordism or post-Fordism is an empirical question, with no theological answer.

The funding of health services (ability and willingness to pay for public services, on the part of different socio-economic classes and strata, and the dependence of such willingness upon the distribution of benefit) is affected by the changing distribution of income and effort in the economy as a whole. If the latter is post-Fordist, there will be an effect upon health services 'internally' as well. Additionally, the benefits offered through public NHSs et al may be subject to change – as the state 'uses' the NHS as part of its 'social investment' mission, either through a 'functionalist' steering to preserve economic competitiveness or through 'instrumental' control of the state by a different coalition of social classes, interests and groupings. And of course differentiated 'post-Fordist' workforces may reflect both the need to recruit and retain as well as the need to maximise output/exploitation.

Yet in other cases, this may best be done by mass workforces (if you like, mirroring the earlier stage of Keynesianism when 'wage creep' and the politics of incomes policies had not yet lowered profits and/or retarded aspirations for higher wages on the part of skilled workers.) In the NHS furthermore 'higher wages for higher skills' had always applied, but on the basis of guilds and not necessarily related to productivity or 'output-based' criteria as opposed to input-based trade union bargaining under Whitley Councils.

Looking at the macro-economy in the UK, Mrs Thatcher 'sold herself' to skilled workers at the core of the economy (in 1979) – ironically as an alternative to incomes policies which were more egalitarian (within the working class, not across society) and therefore unappealing to core workers beneath the level of rhetoric ('Socialism is about equality; trade unionism is about differentials'...to which one might add, 'and individualism is about what you can get, either through productivity or through industrial muscle even if the latter uses collectivist rhetoric.') Yet the reality was that higher incomes had to be earned through vastly greater productivity – not through 'holding the government to ransom, the approach tried under old Labour, which did not work even when it worked, in that it produced a marginally larger share of a smaller cake.

The question for even the 'core' workers is: do you want a little more for a lot of extra work/intensity, or do you want equity at the expense of 'competitive efficiency'? Within the NHS, the same question applies when 'reprofiling' workforces and 'upskilling' etc.

Indeed the transition from what Jessop calls the Keynesian Welfare National State (KWNS) to what he calls the Schumpeterian Workfare Postnational Regime

(SWPR) can be considered in terms of this choice, to remove some of the overtones of determinism (not that such choices are easy, easy to offer or even easy to formulate in the global capitalist environment).

The KWNS sought full employment – as the basis of citizenship but more fundamentally as the means of creating adequate demand/consumption in the capitalist economy – that is why the characterisation is Marxist. Additionally the state provided social investment, i.e. infrastructure for private capitalism of the sort it was unwilling (the problem of collective action) or unable (due to 'zero profits under perfect competition) to provide.

Regarding (5) above: under perfect competition, the only way firms can produce profit is through exploitation i.e. the extraction of surplus value. This is the sense in which Marx both started with and then extended classical economic theory. But under the KWNS, workers could get their full dessert – for two reasons. Firstly, full employment increased their bargaining power; and, secondly, the key industrial sectors were monopolistic or oligopolistic, with the result that firms profits came from pricing policy to consumers. Now these consumers were also workers, so the rewards to capital and labour could be relatively the same as when perfect competition plus exploitation applies. That is, workers would 'get more but also pay more.'

Of course the prevailing political coalitions may have tipped power in the direction of labour, through both taxation policy and direct control of industry. This is broadly what happened. And (therefore) another difference is that, under the KWNS, the work/leisure balance was different; and there was (a lot) less work/intensity for a bit less income (as the economy's full productive capacity was lower than it could be, under deliberate, nationally-controlled industrial and economic policy).

At the level of the regime of accumulation (in the language of regulation theory), all this changed as a response to 'crisis (both objective and discursive/linguistic), which resulted in political action to reflect the electoral coalition's (and the dominant business interests') reaction to the alternatives i.e. the 'Keynesian plus' alternative economic strategy (Benn, 1989) (never properly articulated for the electorate and/ or hegemonic within the Labour party, despite the campaigns of leftists such as Tony Benn); 'more of the same' i.e. reluctant retrenchment under Labour; and the reinvigoration of capitalism under Thatcher. And the rest is history.

Hence regarding (4) above, the Thatcherite strategy both responded to and further caused the internationalisation of capitalism and the reliance upon international business as part of the accumulation strategy.

The question now for health services is: does the NHS mirror the economy? Up to a point, but only up to a point (the wider economy is 'post-Fordist because of the interplay between the changed structure of demand and the changed organisation of and rewards to production and employment ...as well as changing technologies and power relations in supply. This is less true in the NHS.) Regarding (4) above, as already noted, there are various ideologies around to 'justify' new trends, policies and management approaches – and these vary from the collectivist to the individualist (e.g. pay and 'human resources' policy is a compromise between the national or 'equitable' and the local or 'efficient'/''incentivised').

The NHS is Fordist but is now abolishing 'guilds' and Trade Union-based differentials in the labour force (e.g. through Agenda for Change) and the separate deals for different cadres of worker which characterised the epoch – but not the logic – of Fordism.

Thus, regarding (6) and (7) above: which we have not yet overtly discussed, the move to regime governance in the NHS is vastly overrated, and indeed dependent upon believing the rhetoric behind policy (itself devised for political enemies rather than to plan a new approach.) And, the means by which any 'post-Fordist' NHS would be legitimated or accepted is as yet unclear – it is rejected by most cadres of the medical profession (albeit for a mixture of altruistic, economic and atavistic reasons) and rejected also by the public (except when immediate need puts consumerism above citizenship). Its acceptance is greatest ironically among less privileged professionals who see an opportunity for greater responsibility. Yet low-skilled workers, ironically, tend to lose out under 'post-Fordism'.

It is worth keeping in mind that to characterise the move from Keynesian demand management and (possibly) social democracy to 'post-Fordist' supply-side economics as regime change may be over-egging the pudding. Even neo-classical economists, never mind Keynesians, see the 'Marxist' argument for managing demand and investing in social infrastructure. Keynesian demand management may be mirrored rather than rejected by 'supply-side' investment – the difference then is in the distribution of income and wealth (Ronald Reagan, the supply-side President was a kind of super-Keynesian of a regressive sort). The key issue is globalisation or at least internationalisation: how compelling (and how monolithic) is it?

Regarding (4) – the pivotal level of the state – we may consider the European Union. EU health **services** policy is currently conspicuous by its absence or peripheral nature. EU policy-makers assume that, by eschewing health services policy, they can leave national health policy regimes to incremental change, distant from the EU single market et al. Yet the single market deeply affects the 'stuff' of health services (i.e. labour; consumers; capital; goods and services. (Paton et al, 2001) And the trend therefore is to competition at least within a widened Europe, perhaps in the context of fiscal restraint in public health services as a result of EU macro-economic and fiscal policy. This accentuates the reality that Europe's pre-Fordist health systems (e.g. the guilds of Germany, both in insurance and in supply, and the politically-connected interest coalitions of France) are structurally suitable for post-Fordist implementation – even when it might be rational to construct (structurally) Fordist healthcare systems within post-Fordist economies for various reasons (consider the case of France, trying to solve some of its healthcare excesses by moving in a Beveridge direction; and see Part 3 of this paper above).

Let us now look more carefully at the NHS.

The Underlying Causes of 'The NHS Problem'

So, if the NHS exhibits characteristics of 'plus ça change', why is it in crisis? Proponents of the theory of 'fiscal crisis' in the 1970s (such as James O'Connor (1973) and Ian Gough (1979)) argued that the state could not spend enough to provide economic and social infrastructure and social legitimacy while keeping taxation and regulation at a low enough level to allow capitalism to flourish (Bacon and Eltis, 1976, mirrored this argument, from the Right). By the 1980s, the Right's response was to go for the latter while reshaping society (ideologically as well as economically) to change expectations in the former realm.

For the NHS, this created a paradox. It had to become **so** efficient by comparison with alternatives (including the private sector) that citizens (voters) prioritising lower taxes above more welfare would still 'buy into' it economically as well as culturally. That is, in paying taxes for the NHS to include their own needs but also some limited redistribution to the poorer, they would still get a better deal than in making their own private arrangements. The question for the NHS, despite all the rhetoric from the right-wing think tanks and the Sunday papers, was: can it provide so much more bang for the buck than alternatives that it can both distribute according to expectations and redistribute as well, for the same money 'per middle England capita.' And therein lay the rub: in order to do this, it had to be a clinically sound but cheap and (not so) cheerful service, based upon Fordist production lines in a post-Fordist age. And so – culturally rather than economically; in terms of quality of hotel services and waiting lists – the NHS became less attractive to the better-off, despite its best efforts – a victim of its own success.

Klein (2002), Moran (1999) and Salter (1998) have all in various ways written on the unwritten bargain between the state and the medical profession which kept the state out of (the) surgery and doctors out of parliament. This required a public which accepted medical wisdom and both a Ford rather than Rolls Royce service and also prevailing modes of informal rationing, keeping such decisions as 'low politics'. When the economic, political, and cultural underpinnings of this acceptance broke down, the state blamed the doctors and the doctors blamed the state. We don't need soul-searching facilitated seminars to probe low morale in the medical profession – it's the (political) economy, stupid.

To ask a related question: why was the most cost-effective health care system in OECD Europe subjected to the most (arguably) radical, (undeniably) persistent and escalating reform from the 1980s onwards? Either the forces pushing reform were more than cost-related or governments were characterized by a mixture of stupidity and the perceived need to indulge in symbolic politics with electorates...or blinded by ideology of the wrong sort!

Indeed there is a paradox at the heart of the Beveridge system which goes back to the original Beveridge approach to the welfare state. This was to provide a universal minimum (stress on the latter), although clearly, of the 'five giants', health and education were to be more comprehensively funded than social assistance, unemployment benefit and housing. 'Writing in' progressive (as opposed to flat) financing, generous entitlements and building in the whole population to social benefits such as SERPS (the State Earnings-Related Pension Scheme) was always a challenge, and always the part of the Beveridge settlement most under threat. In an age of greater inequality, keeping health care both universal and comprehensive is likewise a challenge, not because of the efficiency or otherwise of the NHS but because of political economy and the dominant ideology of welfare (amongst policy-makers rather than – just – the public.) (Taylor-Gooby,1985)

To put it another way, post-Fordism is neither new nor 'post' anything as far as the welfare state is concerned!

The big questions now are: *firstly* (even if the government's laudable spending plans for the NHS survive the trade cycle over the next five or six years) whether current sources of extra revenue can be extended to 2020 in line with the recommendations to the British Chancellor of Derek Wanless (even on the least expensive of his three scenarios); and *secondly*, whether the state and the doctors can repair their relationship on a new basis; and whether 'reform' to the NHS provides real improvements.

Answering the first question to the benefit of the NHS requires willingness to pay by electoral majorities, and probably altruism or solidarity as well as self-interest on the part of swing voters (in the absence of radical change to national and international political economy which leads to a society stressing lower cash income in return for more leisure and greater sustainability. Currently swing voters work a lot harder for a little extra disposable income, by comparison with the 1970s, for example).

Doctors and the State ...

Regarding the second question above: the unwritten, informal deal between the state and doctors meant that the doctors did not seriously question overall resources or their public-sector pay, and therefore were left alone to 'do the rationing' their way. They did it in the context of professional and clinical autonomy (and also liberal private sector opportunities for some specialties because of a vaguely written public (NHS) contract. The new contracts for doctors from 2004 were geared to reversing this informal deal: doctors would get more money in return for less autonomy. The sources of diminished autonomy are of course multiple, not least public expectations.

Paradoxically, when money was tighter in the 'old NHS', although autonomy for the profession was the price of underfunding at the level of the political 'deal', underfunding meant that 'autonomy' (ie difficult rationing decisions) could be burdensome (even 'doing the rationing our own way' was becoming irksome for the doctors). Yet governments needed doctors to have enough autonomy so that tough decisions were not placed politically at government's door, either by doctors or the public. Thus doctors, having wanted autonomy in theory, might be disillusioned with its implications in practice. Governments paradoxically however rely on (partial) medical autonomy, and abolish it at their peril.

The 'new devolution' in the NHS (DoH, 2001) spoke with a forked tongue. It promised to empower doctors at the front line yet did so by co-opting them. And it meant the state saying to the doctors, 'we know your autonomy is diminished, and that our reforms will diminish it further. In return, we'll pay you'. More money for doctors meant a recognition of less medical autonomy, and the government had lost the political advantage of the doctors carrying, or at least sharing, the burden of tough decisions.

The trouble by 2006 furthermore was that the changed 'quid pro quo' (less autonomy, more money) was becoming unaffordable: despite new money for the NHS, higher productivity (more operations) by better paid doctors was being restricted, to solve deficits! And in primary care, the GPs had been paid lots in return for very little. The public (rightly) blamed the government for 'botching' the NHS's new pay arrangements. Furthermore, since doctor's priorities were now transparently set by the state, the public also (rightly) blamed the government for both the consequences of rationing and the phenomenon of 'post-code healthcare'.

... Doctors and Political Economy

In the early NHS, the policy was universalism and comprehensiveness; and both limited technology and political economy allowed this part-laudable fact, part-fiction to apply. Medical possibilities were more limited; and in terms of political economy we were in the era of the industrial welfare state. As a result, the state did not have to invest selectively in niche industries and services to ensure international competitiveness. The welfare state helped capitalism reproduce itself through social investment, to be distinguished from social expenses (O'Connor, 1973.) That was chickenfeed compared to today's 'competition state' which makes the state less autonomous, less a guarantor of universalism and yet more complex in its economic role.

What rationing was necessary was done informally, by doctors acting within the state's distribution of resources (both primary and specialised ... for example, GPs would 'turn away' the elderly for kidney transplants by custom and practice; or would turn away those for whom hospital referral was a tall order due to local lack of provisions, unsuitability for travel *et al.*)

That is, implementing policy fitted in with the unwritten grand design of policy – the noble lie, if you like.

Nowadays, the policy is both to invest in the (capitalist) economy in the context of global capitalism, and to ensure responses to consumerism and demands for higher quality, by no means just by the middle-classes, although more by them. This necessitates more money and more intensive use of resources including human i.e. 'exploitation' to increase economy-wide returns by squeezing more from workers.

Consider the hypothesis discussed above that state-funded health services (such as the NHS) are a cheap means of investment in the workforce and the economy. If firms derive extra profit (surplus value) as a result of healthier workers which is due to social spending, then that extra profit can be defined of as the total extra income minus the costs of the social spending (e.g. corporate tax used to contribute to the NHS) which firms make. The residual – the extra profit – is composed of two elements – the contribution which workers make to their own healthcare costs and social expenses (e.g. through tax) which increases their productivity and firms' profits; and the exploitation, i.e. 'surplus value' extracted from, healthcare workers. This latter element, if it exists, derives from the incomes of healthcare workers being less than the value they create i.e. the classic Marxist definition of surplus value.

Implementation of such a strategy means that doctors and others must be 'on board' (as managers would put it) regarding priorities and whom to prioritise... otherwise firms will not get what they need from the NHS and/or the public won't. And if this is so, then either firms will make greater use of private occupational healthcare and/or individuals will use the private sector more. Either way, the tax base of the NHS will be undermined, as firms and individuals are less willing to pay for a service that does not deliver what they want.

And **if** doctors and others are 'on board' with the NHS's mission to invest in the workforce, then poorer (less economically central) strata in society may find that the NHS's relative exit from general care and rescue makes it less appealing to them.

Thus, to have the active support (as opposed to the sullen acquiescence) of the worse-off and less economically productive, the NHS must be fair and universal; to have the support of the middle-classes as consumers, it must be a modern service of three or preferably four-star quality and hotel status; and to have the support of industry, it must provide a healthy workforce at economical cost.

Hence the ambitiousness of the NHS Plan. Perhaps we can describe it as an attempt to preserve social democratic 'Fordism' in a cold climate. Unlike in the rest of the economy, there is a real 'third way', and it is in fact the first way.

PART 2
Public Policy

Chapter 3

Public Policy and the State

Explaining Public Policy

The literature concerning the factors which influence, shape and even 'cause' public policy is now immense. It is necessary to walk the tightrope between theory, on the one hand, and plausible explanation of what is actually happening in the real world, on the other hand. Rhodes (in Stoker (Ed), 2000) stated memorably that social science can cope with a lot of hindsight, a little insight and almost no foresight! Thus it is with explanations of public policy.

The 'policy process' is a phrase which characterises the story of how policies develop; are implemented, in often unpredictable or even perverse ways; amended, in a process which is less linear than (variously) wave-like, stew-like, cyclical and even circular. (Hill, 1997) It should also be understood to encapsulate how politics both shapes and is shaped by policy and the social outcomes which result from policy 'outputs.'

The key factors used in political science and public administration to explain outputs and outcomes in public policy are:

(1) political economy (generally, and also embracing 'regime' or 'regulation' theory) (Aglietta; 1979; Jessop, 2002). Part 1 above illustrated how political economy is a crucial backdrop to understanding the underlying pressures and constraints upon health policy.

(2) socio-economic factors. These are distinguished from (1) – although related – in that they refer to 'data and demographics', such as the level of wealth of a country and the distribution of wealth and income. Health and welfare expenditure for example has been correlated to the former.

(3) institutionalist, 'new institutionalist' and structural explanations, which give primacy to the effect of political institutions (and the behaviour and 'incentives' which they create) in explaining policy outputs (see for example Paton (1990).) This raises issues of 'structure versus agency'. That is, do structures independently influence and shape human agency or types of action; or is agency the 'primary' category, with structures – and culture – merely 'congealed' manifestations

of human behaviour which are transitory and changeable through agency. This gets us into deep waters in terms of the philosophy of social science. A belief in the primary of agency may be based on existentialism, which would characterise an individual's absorption into the ethos of prevailing structures and cultures as 'bad faith'. Inversely, a belief in the primacy of structure would depict the opposite camp as 'methodologically individualist', with pejorative overtones, implying that the basis for individuals' agency is determined by social (i.e. structural and cultural) factors. There is a middle way, which argues that individuals may act in groups, or share interests which influence their behaviour (i.e. a denial of methodological individualism in the existentialist sense), yet have goals and objectives which are determined independently of political structures (institutions) and of cultural factors (for example, a putative 'dominant ideology'. Nevertheless, their behaviour is influenced by institutions and the 'incentives' to which the latter give rise, as they seek to achieve their objectives in the most 'rational' manner. This is a version of 'institutional rational choice'.

(4) issues of power, which implies analysis of how power is distributed   in society and within the political system, which influence public policy. For example, is power distributed pluralistically, or are decisions taken by – or in the interests of – (a) ruling elite(s) or even a ruling class? Here, it is important to distinguish instrumentalism (arguing that, if politics and policy benefit a group, elite or class, how this occurs must be actually demonstrated) and functionalism (which implies that 'means which are functional for ends' somehow issue forth.) An example of using functionalism to defend Marxism, for example, was found in Cohen (1978.) A 'strong' variant of functionalism is evolutionism, which draws an analogy with Darwinianism in natural science to imply that the policies which come to dominate are those best suited to surviving in their (political) environment (John, 1999). To me, functionalism implies that policies develop because they are functional for the external environment; whereas evolutionism implies that policies develop if the external environment is functional for them. Neither stance is satisfactory, as the 'how' is missing. And evolutionism in particular – in social science and policy studies – is either tautologous or vacuous. This is because, unlike in the natural world, the 'environment' is man-made and mutable (see 'agency versus structure' above!), and can be 'made' functional for policies. Anything can therefore be explained in this manner.

Network 'theory', whether sociological, political or managerial has had prominence recently (Marsh (Ed.) 1998). To me it is descriptive rather than analytical, although if integrated with 'power studies' (i.e. networks 'explained' in terms of power and influence) could be more powerful itself! It is currently heavily associated with the 'governance' movement (which contrasts the gerundive and vague 'governance' with the traditional and 'reified' government). Empirically it depicts the networks – often bringing together public and private (voluntary, not-for-profit or commercial) actors and agencies – which work together to implement (or even create) policy. As with networks in general, it often 'redescribes' familiar situations in 'social science-ese' without adding insight. At its best however it has the potential to explore how regimes at various levels of government (international, national and local) are responsible for investment and consumption – and therefore to link political economy with institutional and behavioural analysis. For example, the 'corporatist' approach – which depicts 'iron triangles' of business, government and labour in policy decision-making (Cawson, 1982) – was extended to depict how national government organises investment and local government organise consumption. More recently, in the 'global and European' era, local and regional government and governance are responsible for investment to a greater extent, with national government ironically increasingly controlling or circumscribing consumption. This is related to a (concealed) change in power relations in the economy, with corporatist 'tri-lateralism' replaced with the 'bi-lateralism' of business and the state.

(5) 'rational choice theory' – including institutional rational choice theory, introduced above in (3) – has a presence in both economics and politics literatures in the guise of 'maximising behaviour'. It should be distinguished from 'the 'rational actor' perspective in government and public administration, because the 'rational actor' in the sense of Allison (1971) may or may not be a maximiser, and also because Allison's paradigm or lens of the 'rational actor' is a particular perspective which posits a unified (executive) actor in central government. This is different from a scenario of pluralism (whether within the central state; within society; or in state/society relations), in which separate interests are maximisers and yet (indeed therefore) the outcome is a 'log-rolled' compromise in which maximisers 'trade votes' and end up 'satisficing', given the configurations of power they face in the political institutions which they have to use to transact their business.

(6) Ideas and ideologies – which are important, but often linked to wider social factors (and political economy), and in complicated ways. An approach emphasizing the primacy of ideas may sound 'rational.' On the other hand, an approach emphasizing 'ideology' may be ambiguous. Ideology can suggest moral goals and a programme to achieve them…or it can suggest false consciousness of agents as 'cultural dupes.'

Policy in Practice – the Contradictions

The seemingly random interplay of ideas, groups organised around either ideas or interests (or 'advocacy', combining both (Hann, 1995)) and opportunities for policy decisions, leads us to the 'garbage can' approach (Cohen, March and Olsen, 1972) (I apply this approach to New Labour's health policy, below.) Policy now seems an arbitrary mess. And it may be, at one level or for some of the time. The question then arises: how is policy rationalised, if indeed it is, to ensure that the aims of the state are realised? This is a more fundamental question than one about the aims of government. Clearly individual governments' aims simply may not be realised. Not should one assume that there is some teleology or functionalism favouring the 'aims of the state.'

My argument is a different one. Let us illustrate with health policy. I argued above in Part 1 that an institution such as the NHS is only politically legitimate and economically viable if it satisfies several conditions. These are: investment in domestic workers occupying salient niches in the international economy; acceptability to the 'demanding' middle-classes, in terms of both quality and financial outlay (i.e. comparable to what they'd pay if only insuring themselves); and fulfilment of its egalitarian founding mission at least to the extent that it seems worth the moral bothering of protecting in the first place.

How can action by the state or its agents seek to fulfil these conditions? How in other words does the political realm ensure the compatibility of social institutions (such as the NHS) with economic reproduction? There is no inevitability here. If it fails, then these social institutions will be vulnerable. For example: if the NHS does not satisfy employers' needs and demands for healthy employees, employers will seek to finance its own occupational health. If doctors fail to cooperate at least adequately to prioritise the 'outputs and outcomes' which the state requires, then either they will be coerced into so doing within the NHS or they will be disciplined by market forces outside the NHS, as corporations take responsibility for healthcare on a sectional basis (perhaps taking advantage of European Union law.)

What this does, then, is give a government such as New Labour – sympathetic to preserving the NHS means of at least financing healthcare – an interest in ensuring that the state coordinates policy 'at the end of the day', so that a complex amalgam of aims can be furthered. There is in practice a major conflict between the 'post-modern garbage can' of policy initiatives under New Labour and this need for coordination. The latter means tight control of resources given the ambitiousness and complexity of aims – which means political centralism against all prevailing rhetoric. The former however stresses fragmentary 'market' and 'devolving' initiatives, stemming not from evidence about health policy but from both ideological insecurity (fear that the middle-classes will see the NHS as 'Stalinist' in a (post-) Thatcherite age) and the bossy tinkering by natural Fabians thwarted by being born out of time.

The latter is handled, therefore, indirectly: the politicians 'do' the ideology (while denying they are ideological) and a class of political managers does the enforcing, sweeping away the more nonsensical policy contradictions 'in the darkness' once the media has moved on. The problem with the latter approach is that the rationalising is therefore done by the 'faceless bureaucrats': when challenged, whether by MPs or the public, it (deservedly) lacks legitimacy. So the government has to compromise even more, not having had the courage to make hard choices and eschew contradictory policies in the first place; and not having the courage to do its own rationalising in the second place, instead delegating that to 'managers.'

Later in this chapter, I apply the 'garbage can' to New Labour's health policy. Part 3 then explains the detail of that policy, and the means used to 'clean up the garbage' behind the scenes.

Increasingly we can see that, in order to explain public policy outputs, we have to consider, respectively: the backdrop of political economy; social power; the structure of the state and political institutions; and how individuals, groups, interests and classes behave in the context of the structures they must use.

For example, Allison's Model 1 (*op. cit*) posits a unified executive pursuing the 'national good', having been developed 'empirically' to explain the US government's behaviour during the Cuban missile crisis. It is therefore a kind of 'grounded theory' which is context-specific; and therefore the model may be less suitable for wider explanation of social decision-making, interest-group politics and power.

Institutional rational choice theory is an attempt to go beyond the context-specific, but it may be culture-specific. It is useful in that it 'situates' maximising behaviour in an institutional context, and therefore avoids the universal mathematical homilies of neo-classical economics as the root of all politics. It is in principle capable of taking account of structural as well as 'autonomous agency'-type factors (e.g. the kind of institution one is operating from within shapes the incentives and therefore the behaviour). Dowding is right to remind critics that the approach need not be 'methodologically individualist.'

Yet two more fundamental criticisms apply. At the conceptual level, it still posits a version of the 'Modernist Man' which Margaret Archer has gently but scathingly criticised in her latest book (2000), the alternative not being post-modernism but authentic humanity. At the empirical level, its explanations are frequently implausible and indeed 'under-determined' in that the explanandum can be explained much more plausibly and humanly. (See for example James, 1995). Just as many post-modernist 'management theorists' are philosophers-manques, it seems that many 'rational choice' political scientists are motivated by 'showing their macho' in the disciplinary struggle for hegemony with economics!

To me, the challenge is to incorporate different explanatory factors at different levels of analysis. These levels can be considered to be a hierarchy in that there is a move from the 'underlying' to the 'immediate' in terms of their causal nature as regards policy outputs, but this is heuristic rather than wholly empirical. It is important not to be too rigid about (for example) what is undoubtedly a two-way relationship between political structure and social power: the latter will exert itself, except in exceptional circumstances, through different forms of structure, it is true; but the former's mode of channelling power may alter the nature of that power in so doing.

For example: the medical profession was powerful, as a stratum within a social and economic elite in the thirty post-war years of the last century, in both the UK and USA. It was capable of exerting its power through the then-very different political institutions of the UK and the USA. In the centralised, executive-heavy UK with (then) a political culture of insider networks which were relatively invisible (like all effective power!), an implicit bargain was made through informal channels between the state and the profession, which meant a symbiotic relationship in governing the NHS. In the US, with its decentralized interest-group politics as the 'stuff' of the system, the profession preserved its power using different institutions in different ways – primarily by blocking reform (in the way that the insurance industry did with the Clinton Plan in the 1990s, by which time it had replaced the now 'toothless tiger' of the American Medical Association (AMA) as the lobby feared by reforming legislators).

The question which arises is: is power economically-rooted at base, with the decline in the AMA's – and wider medical profession's – power caused by a surplus of doctors, on the one hand, by comparison with the 1950s and 1960s (when access to healthcare was extended by government, and the medical profession's fears of 'socialisation' were shown to be ideological rather than economic!), and by new corporate approaches to purchasing and organising health care for their workers, on the other hand?

There is clearly truth in this. Yet it is not the whole story. The centralist UK political system was capable of more systematic reform – including the creation of the NHS itself – than in the US, when the state was governed by a strong political party with clear and comprehensive aims – in other words, 'majority rule' rather than the passage of policy by the painstaking assemblage of winning coalitions in the legislature. The latter creates a 'mobilisation of bias' (Schattschneider, 1960) away from comprehensive or 'rationalist' reform as opposed to incremental reform, which in turn alters mindsets and limit ambitions (Paton, 1990). That is, structures can have cultural and ideological effects.

Admittedly one can argue that, in Britain, the executive culture of the time (of insider power, and informal insider networks linking civil servants and the economically powerful) acted as a brake upon radical reform. It did. But this is an example of cultures having structural effects i.e. the opposite to the situation in the US. Where politicians (e.g. the Labour government of 1945 or the Conservative governments after 1979) 'rode out' opposition from elite orthodoxies, policy enactment was possible. It was of course the case that, in the implementation of the enacted policy to create an NHS, elites could seek to recoup some of the power which had been overridden at political/policy level. But arguably a 'bias had been mobilised' which – in the long term – created a 'path dependency' which allowed more equitable national health policy.

It is important however not to 'reify' political structures and institutions so that the analyst is blinded to their different use in different eras or under different 'regimes' in political economy. In the heyday of the **national** state, it is not surprising that variation between nations as to political structure and institutions was more significant in producing and explaining policy variance. The story I told in Paton (1990) about how US political structures created a mobilisation of bias away from equitable and comprehensive health reform is one I stand by. But it is a story of its time, although still with insight for understanding US institutions (see for example

Mann and Ornstein (Eds.), 1995) The UK was the implicit alternative model, in the story I told, with the relative autonomy of its central state by comparison with the US: radical reform against elite interests was more possible. Yet today, especially for countries such as the UK where the 'domestic market' is less self-contained than in the US, political institutions per se are less significant in an age of capitalist globalisation than in the period about which I was writing.

Paradoxically we see more policy 'hyper-activism' in England (I talk of England, post-devolution within the UK after 1999) today than ten, twenty and certainly thirty years ago. But this is in part 'a raging at the fading of the light', as well as the post-modern pathology of political itchy-fingers in an era of political amnesia and solipsism as well as media-induced grasshopper-minds on the part of the citizenry.

It is important to study an issue such as health policy over a long enough period (subjectively, about twenty to thirty years, in today's world) to allow different eras to 'register' and therefore to perceive the changing salience of different explanatory factors in public policy. In a nutshell, the 1970s were the era of 'political structures', as the prevailing political economy **was** nationally-based; the 2000s are the era of political economy, as capitalist globalism reduces the salience of nations and their institutions. When I examine New Labour's health policy, below, in terms of policy hyper-activism and governmental 'itchy fingers', the resultant policy output is presented as dysfunctional managerially but rooted in the government's desire to 'change cultures', believing that is the price of (for example) the NHS's survival.

In other words, political economy is at the top of the hierarchy of salient factors in delimiting and explaining public policy. It sets the background, environment and constraints. Depicting a regime in political economy shows how the state and other elements of the polity 'come together' to steer the economy in a particular way. It is Marxisant, in that it prioritises 'economic production', situates political viability and legitimacy in terms of the political economy and has 'crisis' as the motivation to move from one type of regime to another (for example, from the Keynesian national welfare state to the Schumpeterian workfare state, in the language of Jessop (2002). It is however post-Marxist or non-Marxist in that regimes vary within capitalism: that is, a regime is less than a mode of production in the Marxist sense.

Institutions and political structures shape behaviour – partly by channelling 'rational' behaviour (i.e. 'institutional rational choice') but also by changing cultures and expectations, which feed into future 'ideas' for policy, reform or whatever, as outlined above.

Power is exerted, that is, through institutions overtly and covertly, but the latter equates neither to Lukes nor to the post –structuralist vision of dialogues which are enclosed even if arbitrary (unlike their structuralist progenitors.) Loss of ambition in reform ideas is a fatalism, in this sense, rather than a false consciousness, perhaps because elites are 'systematically lucky' (in Dowding's arresting oxymoron which in the end is just that...an oxymoron, because – with reflexivity of actors and even of 'passive' public(s) – those who are systematically lucky are likely to go beyond luck i.e. to build on initial luck in order to make deliberate strategy).

Political structures/institutions vary between countries (as well as sub and supra-national levels). Thus executives vary in structure, scope, salience and power, within the political system in general and state in particular (Regimes are more than governments and less than state systems – they are means of using state systems and structures to achieve ends through means which transcend e.g. 'party competition')

Ideas (and ideologies, whether or not recognised as such in an age which is coy about 1970s terms!) seem increasingly influential in policy – whether it is the 'cultural imperative' of introducing consumerism and choice into the NHS, for example, or the persistent re-organisations in response to 'bright ideas' whether from academics or management consultants. We must distinguish the two levels.

The first – culture/ideology – I consider to be rooted in political economy. It would be perfectly possible to debunk the shortcomings of the 'choice' model in an era when the 'majority' electoral and political coalition did not depend upon pleasing a consumerist stratum of 'swing voters.' At the very least, the cultural and the economic are mutually-embedded: the growth of the 'demanding consumer' is not part of a historical law distinct from consideration of economic regimes.

The second level – embodied in 're-organisations' – is different. These are an 'autonomous' distraction – autonomous but 'trivial' in the sense that the garbage-can which produces them (see below) must be periodically cleansed. If they are dysfunctional for the state's objectives as pursued by the governing party, they will be marginalized, if not reversed, 'behind the scenes.' That is why those who defend a market approach to the NHS, for example, are wrong to see its marginalisation as a 'betrayal' by statist civil servants or the like. It is less than that, or rather more than that. It is an attempt to reconcile policy – undertaken not by traditional civil servants but by 'meso'-level political managers between the centre and 'the field.' The traditional civil servants, for their part, are doing traditional things – for example, devising systems to implement strands of policy (such as the 'choice policy'; the 'specialised services policy'; the 'targets policy')…'down silos' without reference to what is happening in the next room at Richmond House, the Department of Health's HQ. For a government which made 'joined up policy' both a mantra and a piece of jargon, New Labour's domestic policy-making is the least joined-up of all post-war governments.

Politicians blame 'traditional' civil servants for acting as a brake upon policy (Blair every bit as much as Thatcher). And civil servants are often intelligent amateurs who 'pigeon hole' policies and implement the letter but not the spirit of reforms (eg 'Choose and Book' in the NHS). Yet it is political amateurism which fails to go beyond 'policy consumption' as an end in itself to effective reconciliation of different objectives – and thus aids the 'pigeon holing'.

The Metaphor of the 'Garbage Can'

The garbage can is the metaphor originally used by Cohen, March and Olsen (*op. cit*) to refer to a non-rational – if not arbitrary – decision-making process in organisations (actually a university, in the original article). To adapt their elegant work: when it is perceived that there is an opportunity for influencing or making a decision i.e. when a 'decision point' is emerging for whatever reason, everyone with an interest in the process brings along their baggage – or 'garbage'. The decision which emerges from the can is not 'rational' (defined as the best decision to relate 'means' to 'ends'), for reasons discussed below.

Political science has analysed for decades the interplay of interests, 'networks', elites and the (resulting) operation of power in allegedly 'pluralist' political systems. There are many models which depict how multiple interests 'battle it out', with policy outcomes often pleasing none of the interests involved – perhaps consisting in the 'lowest common denominator' to allow enactment of the policy. Alternatively the model of 'log-rolling' (or vote trading) depicts how all participants in the legislative process can be pleased, but at the expense of the polity or economy (usually in terms of the costs to be borne).

Political scientists and students of public administration have predictably extended and applied the 'garbage can' approach to the public policy process. A notable example is Kingdon (1984). His variant of the 'garbage can' approach to explaining public policy involves three elements of the policy process – problems, policies, and politics. These are seen as rival 'streams' which are independent of each other. When they meet, that is the 'decision point' i.e. the place at which policy is likely to be made; at which action happens. Agendas do not necessarily lead to action. And when they do, it may not be the 'agenda-setter' who wins. Kingdon's examples are mainly from US politics, and indeed health policy features strongly. The issue therefore arises as to whether the 'culture' of the model is American rather than universal. For example, an important empirical conclusion, drawn from Kingdon and used by Mann and Ornstein (Eds, 1995) in analysing the Clinton proposals for health reform in 1993-4, is that the President is usually the agenda-setter but equally usually the loser in the legislative fight.

An important question is whether the 'garbage can' approach adds much to the more conventional models of compromise and log-rolling. I think it did, and does – but to me the operative word is 'add': that is, the approach is a supplement or complement rather than a substitute. Explaining policy in the spirit of the 'garbage can' imputes non-rationality to the order in which different 'streams'– such as Kingdon's policy, politics and problems or issues – are treated in the evolution of actual policy enactments. Which problems are analysed (when they are) is not 'rational' either; neither is the sifting of policy options. 'Politics' clearly may have its own rationality, whether recognisable as such by boffins and rationalists, but its influence in the evolution and enactment of policy is not rational by the definition I offer as relevant to public policy i.e. defining and agreeing 'ends' and selecting evidence-based (or at least judgementally appropriate) 'means' to achieve these.

Rationality, Irrationality and the Nature of Policy

The question of whose rationality is of course a basic and familiar one. Unless all values or goals are shared (and in the same proportions to boot (Gray, 1995)) then the pursuit of ends 'rationally' will still result in a pluralistic polity where rival goals have to be mediated politically. This may produce incrementalism in policy-making not because of Graham Allison's (1971)'Model 2', in which conservative civil servants control the process and make only minor adjustments, but because the compromise which emerges through pluralism is a 'second best' for all actors with power in the process.

Perhaps the most important respect in which an 'interest-based' or at least 'political bargaining' model (Allison's (1971) Model 3) can be supplemented by the 'garbage can' can be explained as follows. At one extreme, admittedly, the garbage can may simply depict clashing interests, or at least goals, and the exertion of power in their resolution…but power disguised as 'non-rationality' or even anarchy. At the other extreme, however, the garbage can model may be implying that – even at the level of **each** interest/group, never mind the resolution of different interests – the evolution and choice of options is not rational.

In between, we have the view to which I subscribe, which is that the garbage can model is best viewed – empirically, for my purposes in this book – as a 'post-modern' style of politics in a 'late modernist' world in which rationality, indeed cunning, is already needed in order to 'square the circle' of competing demands upon the NHS.

These are not just the traditional pluralist demands: they come from the international economy; from society as a whole, as consumerism takes over; and from different classes and interests within the country as conditioned by the wider environment of the 'post-Fordist' polity. That is, there is already conflict (whether pluralist or not) but the resulting policy tension is exacerbated by a certain arbitrariness in how agendas are mobilised. Yet the resolution of the resulting 'policy anarchy' is vital.

I aim to illustrate this with reference to the raft of health policies under New Labour, between 1997 and 2006, applying the view from the garbage can to individual policies as well as to the manner in which they are combined.

Chapter 4

Illustrating Public Policy – How New Labour Has Made Health Policy

History repeats itself – first time as tragedy; second time as farce

Adapted from Karl Marx

English Politics, Policy and Implementation

Let us start near the beginning. A revealing 'off the cuff' remark from the Chief Executive (at the time) of the NHS in the Department of Health in England (who was a former NHS manager, not a traditional mandarin with a 'sniffy' view about politicians), made in 1998, a year after New Labour had taken office, was that, 'this lot know very little about implementation and aren't interested either.' (1998). The same individual had been in post at the Department of Health since 1993 and had sought to make management sense of the Conservatives' twists and turns in the 1990s. He was a competent and indeed cautious individual, not prone to such remarks; he had long experience of politicians 'making it up as they went along' in policy and implementation. Arguably he should be credited with making as much managerial sense as possible of the Tories' NHS policy between 1993 and 1997. He was speaking with a non-political but deep frustration.

A similar picture – this time after New Labour's first two terms, rather than at the dawn of the Brave New World – comes from the book on education policy written by former Blair adviser on education, Peter Hyman (2005), revealingly titled, '1 Out Of 10: From Downing Street Vision to Classroom Reality.' Hyman is warm about the Blair government, its sincerity and some of its accomplishments. What is more, the ongoing New Labour agenda for education reform arguably has more prospect of success in one respect – schools are less 'interdependent' (despite the worries of Labour opponents of education reform in 2006, including Lady (Estelle) Morris, Education Secretary for part of Labour's second term) than hospitals and the components of the health system. 'Foundation' Schools and the like may represent more genuine 'freedom' than do Foundation hospitals – for 'technical' as well as political reasons. Foundation hospitals may (have to) be controlled more stringently 'within the system': even although this is sometimes presented as external 'regulation', by Monitor, the NHS's 'economic regulator', the reality is very different (see below).

Yet Hyman points out revealingly (pp.384-5): "Politicians are expected to know everything and often act as if they do. Those at the centre relish ideas, and are bored by practicalities. Those who suggest better ways of making policy work are too often dismissed as whingers or as obstructing change...Why can't politicians acknowledge that those on the frontline might know more?...I was someone who loved the big vision and the symbolic policy. Now I realise that real 'delivery' is about the grind, not just the grand..."

To this, I would add that the natural 'brake' on what could be called 'boy scouting' in policy was traditionally provided by the 'Rolls Royce' of the Civil Service. True; this often represented the 'forces of conservatism' (although not intended as the target in Blair's 1999 Labour party conference speech which used that phrase, when Blair cleverly set out how genuinely progressive reforms such as the NHS itself had been opposed by the forces of conservatism then went on to paint the opponents of 'liberal globalisation' as similarly situated). But it also represented (Sir Humphrey jokes notwithstanding), at the best mandarin level, institutional memory, professionalism and stability.

'Teenage scribblers' – advisors from the world of journalese and public relations – and politically-dependent 'new civil servants' have removed the forces of conservatism in government, but have removed the ballast of an 'autonomous state' as well. As a result, the state makes deals with interests from a position of less strength and – arguably – less confidence. Thus we have New Labour's striking combination of arrogance and insecurity.

What Lord Butler (the former Cabinet Secretary who reported on the Blair administration's decision to go to war in Iraq) called, in a different context, 'sofa government' (Meyer, 2005) has doubtless been a cultural preference for the Blair government. The pollsters, the communications chiefs and the party liaison managers have been joined intermittently on Blair's sofa by enthusiastic, bright and arguably schema-driven academics, such as Julian le Grand, who have ideologies to peddle (altruistically and sincerely, for the most part). Ironically they believe themselves to be practical men, recalling Keynes' dictum that, "practical men, believing themselves to be free of all ideological influences, are usually the slaves to some defunct economist."

Yet this cultural preference has been buttressed by other factors, both cultural and structural. Policy has become faster-moving, 'post-modern', if you like; with the government's itchy fingers too keen to pull levers just because they're there, and – to continue the 'post-modern' metaphor, an obsession with the media in a (counter-productive) attempt to keep the attention and approval of a citizenry which has the attention span of a bored gadfly. Britain (now England as regards domestic policy) has the 'fastest law in the West' (Hill, 1997) due to its ever-stronger Executive and a Parliament which – even when it is assertive – is ill-informed (by international comparison), especially with the US Congress, where the problem in domestic policy is the opposite – too much information and analysis, and not enough movement.

Institutional memory is lost at both political and administrative levels. Ministers for the domestic spending Ministries come and go faster than ever; and tend to see even recent history as a foreign country. The mandarin class has both metamorphosed and had to share power with others. It has metamorphosed from a stable block (with disadvantages and advantages) to a more politically-manipulated structure.

For example, Sir Nigel Crisp, the Permanent Secretary (PS) at Health between October 2000 and March 2006 – when he resigned under pressure from Ministers as the NHS financial deficit approached £1 billion – was a former NHS Chief Executive who was designated PS as well as Chief Executive (CE) of the NHS for England. On paper, this looked good. The merging of PS and CE was presented as 'streamlining' by merging two senior posts. Ironically the NHS had developed a Chief Executive separate from the mandarin class headed by the PS following the Griffiths Report in October 1983, which had overtly argued for a management board to 'look down and manage the service' rather than to 'manage up' to politicians as PSs do. (This point had also been made in the early 1980s by the recently-retired PS at Health, Sir Patrick Nairne.)

Reversing it therefore created a potential 'conflict of role' – how could the Minister's aide be the NHS's leader, and vice versa? In practice, the Health PS/ CE has had difficulty in 'speaking truth to power' – telling the various Emperor Milburns and Empress Hewitts (Health Secretaries) that their clothes are at least threadbare! This owes much to the tenure of the 'PS' in Departments such as Health being both short- or fixed-term contract and more politically-controlled than before. Sir Humphrey may have had his disadvantages, but at least he did not owe his position to the patronage of politicians and therefore could speak his mind firmly behind closed doors. Additionally, a Chief Executive who is also PS and has to spend much of his time on the 'Ministerial agenda' is not well-placed to be an inspiring leader of the largest organisation in Europe, with the credibility which comes from being 'an NHS man' rather than 'the Minister's man.'

Being the latter, in an era of policy 'hyper-activism' as under New Labour, makes the job well-nigh impossible – Crisp was a cerebral man of integrity who nevertheless spent much of his time rationalising (to sceptical audiences) the government's ill-thought-out and ill-reconciled strands of policy (see Part 3). 'Special advisers' to the Prime Minister overturned applecarts at a stroke, by-passing both the traditional civil service and expert advisors who actually had experience in running the NHS. Shades of Sir Alan Walters, whose gadfly role had forced Nigel Lawson's resignation as Mrs. Thatcher's Chancellor in 1989. Given the proliferation of the special adviser under New Labour, it is hard now to remember that Labour had criticised the Conservatives in the 1990s for the profusion and cost of 'pointy-head' special advisers. One notable example is the negotiation of new professional contracts – which came back to haunt New Labour in 2005-6. The 'experts' had been both ignored (and removed, in the Gershon 'efficiency review' of 2004-5). Ministers seized control of the process, advised by those who believed that doctors were 'ripping off' the NHS. As a result, the new contract's 'incentives' were more expensive than necessary – based as they were on a perceived need to buy doctors back into the NHS. Yet most were already working beyond contracted hours. And so most doctors were paid more for doing less, as they worked to contract, contributing to the 'crisis of deficits' in 2006.

Political control of 'mandarin' appointments is however not the same thing as the 'autonomous' political agenda crowding out the administrative or managerial. In many cases, New Labour's political and policy stances on health have derived from the 'managerialism' and 'market' approaches which they have absorbed (unwillingly in the case of Dobson, the first Health Secretary and quite willingly after that) from the new style of civil servant and senior NHS executives with an entrée to power. This is especially true when such advice has been necessary to make sense of the 'text-book homilies' presented as policy by the Le Grands (2003) of this world. The power of the civil servants to 'win' should not be overestimated, however: they were a taxi, delivering what had originally been Tory ideas to New Labour's door, rather than an ivory-tower. The era of Sir Humphrey is long gone, across both domestic departments and the Foreign Office. (Meyer, 2005)

In New Labour's early years, Ministers sought to avoid structural reorganisation yet to create a new culture for the NHS, by abolishing the internal market and what Health Secretary Frank Dobson saw as the excessive influence of the business culture. At first his successor Alan Milburn, while moving to a tougher regime of targets, also eschewed 'the new public management', especially in its market form. The central hierarchy he created was not a traditional administrative hierarchy but more in the spirit of 'L'NHS – c'est moi!' We might call this the 'new public administration' rather than the new public management. But this phase soon yielded, in 2002, to more familiar nostrums with which the Conservatives in the 1990s would have been wholly at home.

Indeed New Labour would arguably have benefited from more, not less, political autonomy – to avoid being in thrall to economic orthodoxy which ironically they interpret as exciting modernisation, and to 'public service reform' which sounds managerial but is actually symbolic and even dysfunctional ('Foundation hospitals' et al – see below for a justification of this claim.) Interestingly Hyman (*op. cit* p. 72), on education, argues that, "...the story, contrary to popular myth, of the government has been the depoliticisation of ministers and advisers (who become administrators and managers rather than political advocates), more than the politicisation of the civil service." Hyman argues that the real clash is between fast-moving ministers and advisors working flexibly (images of Health Secretary Alan Milburn bashing out the NHS Plan on his PC at three in the morning) and traditional civil servants. He also argues that when the clash was between the political and the non-political, the civil service "almost always won."

For health, it is more of a mixed picture on the latter point. But when the civil service did win, it was not a victory for coordinated and integrated policy (whether 'conservative' or not) as it might have been in the old days, but for a translation of a 'political policy' (e.g a radical version of patient choice) into an 'administrative silo' which routinised it. This might be because of the traditional civil servant's desire to make it tidy, 'operationalise-able' and 'monitor-able' or because of the former NHS manager's habit of 'managerialising' policy. Recent examples can be found in both the implementation of the Foundation Trust policy and the implementation of patient choice, which has become another bureaucratic silo rather than a real market.

What is missing however is the 'joined up' or integrated health policy – even health system management – that the previous political settlement would have provided, warts and all. It may well be that the old NHS system would not have been wholly sufficient for the stringent economic challenges facing the NHS (i.e. more productivity in the face of a 'multiple agenda', much of it deriving from overall political economy – see Part 1 above.) But the NHS pre-'meddle and muddle' provided significant capacity for effective planning, which baby has been thrown out with the bathwater of 'the forces of conservatism'. In any case, if there was a need to challenge 'consensus management' 1974-style, the Griffiths Report of 1983 provided the means – without the panoply of quasi-market mechanisms, which the late Sir Roy Griffiths (appointed by Mrs. Thatcher to conduct his review) saw as a distraction. It is ironical that politicians (of both main governing parties) have overridden even limited mechanisms to reduce political interference with the management of the NHS, yet set out blueprints for market reforms which require minimal 'politics' if they are to work. (See analysis of 'choice.' in Part 3)

Some of the above can be ascribed to longer-standing explanations – such as the dissonance between the leadership skills required for charismatic leadership of a political party and indeed government, on the one hand, and the skills required to lead complex organizations and enact effective policy, on the other hand. The question arises: has the problem got worse under New Labour? I think that it has, although the trend in that direction predates New Labour; 'itchy fingers' in health reform started under the Conservatives from the 1980s onwards. Nevertheless, we have seen a rising curve under New Labour. The two principle factors making it worse – in health at least – are, respectively, 'policy hyper-activism' by the executive (primarily from the Prime Minister's office) and a change in the structure and culture of government – covering policy advice and administrative support for implementation, on the one hand, and the role of parliament in particular and oversight in general, on the other hand.

Thus we have the irony that a governmental structure in principle quite suitable for 'rational' policy-making (a historically cohesive executive, and a strong executive) has 'undermined itself' through a post-modern culture. Politicians have prioritised the 'initiative' over the genuine innovation, with New Labour Ministers (many of whom have cut their teeth in the parochialism of local government) mistaking ferment for entrepreneurialism. In the US, the downside of pluralism – fragmentation in policy-making, and the undermining of rational planning by vested interests using political niches – is a consequence of the basic political structure. But in England, these features have been a voluntary creation of New Labour's style of government – which has preached modernisation and markets but made a rod for its own back by creating policy, agencies and quangos which 'build in' both public and private vested interests, ranging in the NHS from Patient and Public Involvement Fora (abolished almost as soon as they were created!) through parochial Primary Care Trusts Boards to Private Finance Initiatives and Private/Public Partnerships.

These sound respectively democratic and 'businesslike.' In practice they create both obstacles to efficient decision-making and planning, on the one hand, and private usurpation of public planning, on the other. (See Part 3)

Health Policy Plucked Out of the Garbage Can? – New Labour's Itchy Fingers

Cut to 2006 and the White Paper, Our Health, Our Care, Our Say (DoH, 2006). Ridiculed by Alice Miles in The Times (Feb 1, 2006; p.18), it can also be seen as a case study: in how policy is motivated by the Prime Minister's agenda; is led by the Health Secretary; by-passes elected representatives; is justified in terms of 'public consultation'; rediscovers the obvious; eschews both the 'hard choices' and pre-requisites for effective implementation; and ends up incoherent (to the extent it goes beyond the platitudinous) in that the PM's 'competition' agenda is not abandoned but watered down and rendered both internally inconsistent and inconsistent with other health policies.

Just what are these policies?

In between 1997 and 2006, we have had four major planks of health policy – all pulling in different directions; some but not all capable of being reconciled; and the reconciliation (and abandonment) of policy left to the meso-level 'political managers' in the system.

Stage 1

In 1997, Labour inherits an NHS which it has promised, in the election campaign, to 'save' ('100 days to save the NHS'), yet whose senior managers it has promised not to change much or re-organise. The soundbite is 're-integration without re-organisation.' The new government is pledged to 'abolish the internal market' yet 'retain the purchaser/provider split' (between funding bodies, primarily health authorities, and providers such as hospitals).

The watchword is 'collaboration' within 'local health economies' (they could have been called families, but someone noticed that families are dysfunctional).

In terms of the 'garbage can', let us consider **policy, politics and problems:**

In this case, **policy is politics** (a very French approach, with the French word for policy and politics being the same!). 'We are not the Conservatives' is its main plank. Yet 'abolishing the internal market' is smoke and mirrors: it has already withered on the vine in the Conservatives' last years; 'retaining the purchaser/provider split' is conservatism. We are still at the stage of the 'no policy policy' (to quote Sir Humphrey Appleby from Yes Minister) – which in fact owes its spiritual derivation to Robin Cook's famous remark, when he was Shadow Health Secretary. When an advisor asked Cook in 1990 if he would like him to help develop Labour's health policy, Cook replied by pointing to Labour's popularity with the public on the health issue (about 80% liked Labour's health policy rather than the Conservative government's.) "And that's before we have a policy, so don't you think it might be rather dangerous to develop too much...?"

The **problem** becomes overt in about two years time, in 1999. In 1997, it had existed but was covert, so of little interest to politicians – who tend to believe, with Lord Keynes, that "in the long run we're all dead.". The covert strategic, or underlying, 'problem' was whether or not 'trust' and altruism was an adequate basis for motivating NHS workers; the operational version of this, or immediate problem; was whether or not to retain the apparatus of the 'Thatcher reforms', in particular the 'purchaser/provider split.'

Stage 2

By 1999, the honeymoon was over – for Health Secretary Frank Dobson and for the Labour government. Even the facile 'pledgecard' promise from 1997 to cut waiting **lists** by 100,000 (almost-but-not-quite meaningless without reference to waiting TIMES) was not being met. Productivity was the problem identified by analysts and academics.

A decision-point was looming. Politicians felt they needed to 'do something.' The most enthusiastic proponents of a 'market NHS' (such as the liberal think-tanks, on the 'Right', and Professor Julian le Grand, on the 'Left') had not yet re-grouped after the 'abolition of the internal market' – which ironically was officially accomplished in April 1999 (with the final abolition of GP-fundholding...as if that were the totem of the evil market!), just as angst over NHS stasis was reaching the portals of Downing Street. Another symptom of the garbage can – policies and needs or problems out of time with each other.

Thus the hegemony of the 'market solution' was not yet (re-) established. ('Established' without the 're' is actually correct, in the bigger picture – the Tory policy never achieved hegemony outside the ranks of the more sycophantic NHS managers and chairmen, on the one hand, and the more ingenuous academics, mostly economists, on the other hand, who took the then-government's eulogy of markets at face value). As a result, the Treasury policy of 'central targets' became by default the approach – leading to a command-and-control culture in the NHS which belied the 1997 rhetoric of the 'third way' as applied synthetically to the NHS.

The 'first way' had allegedly been 'hierarchy', from the NHS's beginnings in 1948 up to 1991; the 'second way' was the Tory internal market from 1991-1997; and the third way was to have been local collaboration (sometimes – retrospectively – referred to as the 'networks' approach) without hierarchy or markets! This was spin. For sure, it was possible to depict earlier versions of the NHS as 'centralist' or 'hierarchical'. Yet ironically, from 1948 until the Griffiths reforms of 1983 which introduced general management, the key decision-makers of the time – the doctors – were not really 'on the organisation chart' at all. Thus although one could depict the bureaucratised post-1974 NHS, for example, as a hierarchy form the centre through Regions through Areas down to Districts (and then units i.e. hospitals and so on!) as a hierarchy, this was what Walter Bagehot would have called the 'dignified' rather than 'efficient' part of the constitution! It did not correspond to the real flows of power.

Equally, the market years (which ended about 1995, not 1997) did not mean a reduction in central control but an increase (Paton et al, 1998) And 'the third way' was just rhetoric, at the very least as applied to health – 'local collaboration' was actually centrally-directed 'mandatory collaboration' i.e. an oxymoron.

Thus the High Noon of 'command and control', the Milburn years from 1999 to 2003 (or later) represented a continuation of a trend which had begun innocuously in 1983, been deepened by the Tory 'market' and now was reaching its apotheosis.

This in turn led to problems – targets were discredited by doctors pointing to their perverse effects (and by health executives and some Board Chairmen doing so more privately with Ministers). The 'purchaser/provider split' had been re-named the 'commissioner/provider separation' (in the years when market linguistics were taboo, with a senior NHS Chief Executive – eager to show off his insider credentials – saying without intended humour in 1997, 'Purchasing's out; commissioning's in....but we don't know what it is yet')! Yet different targets were now applied to commissioners and providers, which made the 'split' almost as acrimonious as it had been in the Tory years. At one level, having different targets was understandable i.e. 'health and population targets for purchasers/commissioner; delivery targets for providers such as hospitals. But the failure to 'own them jointly' was the problem, when the inevitable conflict arose over resources – especially before the NHS Plan of 2000 and the subsequent 'Wanless money' after 2002, which increased resources for the NHS. Up until then Labour had deliberately stuck to the Conservatives spending plans as a badge of honour with the City (although the Conservative Chancellor from 1993 to 1997, Kenneth Clarke, pointed out jovially that there was no way he would have stuck to his own targets.

Stage 3

On May 1st, 2001, Health Secretary Alan Milburn appeared at a press conference, flanked by the Director of the new 'Modernisation Agency' (created to lead service reform then abolished two years later by John Reid, Milburn's successor). Milburn announced the appointment and then news of possibly the most ill-fated and ill thought-out of all New Labour's many health service reorganisations, entitled 'Shifting the Balance of Power.' (Note the 'iron law of NHS re-organisation' starting in 1983 with the Griffiths reforms : 'the more change is denied to involve cumbersome structural re-organisation, the more it does.')

It was to be the following year that the 'new market' was heralded. For now, Shifting the Balance of Power – known throughout the NHS as 'StBoP – heralded the radical devolution of commissioning/purchasing from Health Authorities to Primary Care Trusts, almost at a stroke; and the replacement of the eight English regions with 29 'Strategic Health Authorities.'(SHAs) The reason? The official aim was to 'devolve services to the frontline'. This meant involving the GPs and other clinicians, who were on the Boards of Primary Care Groups (the PCTs' predecessors) in mostly advisory roles to the Health Authority, in commissioning across the whole NHS. In practice, of course, it did not work out like that. The creation of statutory Boards for the PCTs – necessary to govern their new pivotal role – actually marginalised doctors by relegating them from the main Board to a 'PEC' (Professional Executive Committee.) A similar irony had occurred with the Conservatives' creation of hospital Trusts in 1991 (advertised as allowing more involvement in management by doctors – but, as in the famous example of Guy's Hospital in London, often relegating doctor-led management Boards.)

What did happen was that myriads of new bureaucracies were created. This was bad enough in itself, but it also meant that 'commissioning' became a local lottery and that service planning for area populations fell through the cracks (a problem in the early years of the Tory market; worse now) (See Part 3).

Incredibly, the real reason for StBoP was to 'dish the opposition'. Ministers had wind of an impending promise by Liam Fox that the Conservatives would 'abolish health authorities' (a general election was due in late spring or summer, 2001). This sounded 'anti-bureaucratic' although was just a symbolic promise. So New Labour – despite having a parliamentary majority of nearly 200 – had to get in first with the politics of pre-emption and rebuttal, and announce its own 'anti-bureaucratic reform' of abolishing the existing 100 health authorities. Thus it was that the most bureaucratic reform yet was born – with more than 400 PCTs replacing 100 Health Authorities (and new 'vested interests' created which obviated rational planning – see below) and 29 new 'Strategic Health Authorities created to replace 8 Regions.

Two years later, both the prevailing structure of PCTs and the SHAs were acknowledged by the Department of Health to be 'not fit for purpose.' The wink was tipped via SHAs to frustrated hospital Trusts – who saw their ability to plan for the future removed – that after the 2005 general election, further re-organisation would occur. In 2006, a watered-down version occurred (with Ministers dissembling that they only reluctantly decided this after the 2005 election) (See Stage 5, below).

Equally incredibly, it was only nine months later that another major change in emphasis occurred – see Stage 4 immediately below. For even in 2001, the official line was that PCTs and hospital Trusts would be local collaborators rather than market actors.

Stage 4

Another decision-point loomed by 2002. This time, the 'market solutions' were on offer, having been refreshed and – to be fair – re-invented in an attempt to take account of some of the flaws in the 'internal market' policy. In February 2002, a slim but seminal paper was issued by the Department of Health – 'The NHS Plan. Next Steps for Investment; Next Steps for Reform." (As with the Conservatives' market reforms beginning in 1989 with the White Paper, Working for Patients, and a related series of Working Papers, reform and associated re-organisation was informally organised but perpetual).

In Labour's new market (see Part 3 below), instead of price competition, prices were to be fixed, through a national tariff with minor regional adjustments and paid to providers according to their workload ('payment by results') – an aspiration of the Conservatives' market in the early 1990s which had never happened – and competition was to be on the basis of quality (See Part 3.) Related, and more radically, 'patient choice' rather than 'purchaser choice' was to drive (what was not, at first, officially called) the 'new market.' (Subsequently it has come to be called that…New Labour can never resist a 'new' prefix!) Part 3 analyses the 'pro' and 'cons' of both the old and new NHS markets, and also what the alternative might be – in order to understand the trend of New Labour's health policy (i.e. a political explanation) and its likely consequences for healthcare (i.e. an analytical explanation).

For now, we can note that, as ever, the market was not to be what it seemed. The story was to be one of choice and paying providers 'by results', but the reality was to be Strategic Health Authorities (merged in 2006 to become Regions again in all but name: see Stage 5 below) and Monitor, the NHS's 'economic regulator', calling the shots. For example, if PCTs could not afford to pay hospitals what they were owed, SHAs gave instructions as to the compromise.

The press and public believed that hospitals were 'holding PCTs over a barrel', playing games to inflate their income. The reality was the opposite: many hospitals were flooded with emergencies which PCTs were not handling in primary care, and also with 'elective' cases which both PCTs and SHAs insisted should be treated to meet government targets – yet for which proper reimbursement was not forthcoming. On paper, therefore, 'payment by results' was good news for busy hospitals. But in practice, both the tariff itself (prices paid for items of healthcare) and its mode of introduction was manipulated. For example, when it was found to be unaffordable to pay hospitals according to tariff, the prices for unanticipated emergency cases were simply halved for Financial Year 2005-6.

Choice was allegedly 'chosen' by the public, in a series of consultations from the DoH. This is rather fatuous, however: we all know opinion polls can produce whatever result is required. There was not – nor could there reasonably have been – any attempt to situate choice in the complex policy environment of 'trade offs' when reaching this result. (For example, how do you ask the public to 'trade off' choice per se – as an end, not a means – and the coherent regional provision of specialised and emergency services?) (See Part 3).

For now, however, the issue is that 'the problem' was met by the politics of 'radical reform' and by the policy of 'patient choice': the three streams came together in a manner which had not occurred in 1997 or 2000, for reasons which neither 'rationality' nor 'evidence-based analysis' can explain.

Stage 5

By Summer 2005, there was (rightly) seen to be a dissonance between the new 'choice' policy and prevailing health agencies – many of which, most notably the Primary Care Trusts (PCTs), had only been created a year or two previously. (Indeed New Labour excelled itself in amateur-ish institution-mongering – in the bossy Milburn years, agencies were conjured up as if there were no tomorrow (for many, there wasn't)! Some were quickly abolished as Milburn's successor as Health Secretary John Reid made his contribution to the Chancellor's Gershon review of 'waste' in government A record was created when one agency was actually abolished before it had found premises for its headquarters; and the National Forum for Patient and Public Involvement (PPI) was summarily axed leaving the local PPI Fora without a coherent mission (a fact painfully all-too-obvious to most who had to deal with them.) For, just as agencies sprout irrationally, 'waste-busting' is often handled irrationally too – as with the cuts in the Department of Health's central staff which removed expertise in implementing the new contract for hospital consultants, which also became painfully obvious.

'Commissioning a Patient-Led NHS' was therefore rushed out in the quiet period, in summer 2005. (See Part 3) It sought to make PCTs larger and more 'strategic', as their detailed role was less necessary given the 'devolution' of choice of provider to patients and what was left of 'commissioning' (still a usefully ambiguous term) allegedly to GP practices. PCTs were also to lose their 'provider' function, as a market approach to the NHS would imply there was a conflict of interest between a PCT buying services from itself.

Ironically, this paper, produced by NHS Chief Executive and Departmental Permanent Secretary Nigel Crisp, and the new Secretary of State Patricia Hewitt, was if anything a deadly combination of the 'rational' and the tacit, although it was unclear why it was the provider role rather than the commissioner role of PCTs which should be abolished. It offended lots of the newly-created interests and fiefdoms (see below). The garbage-can was soon therefore re-opened: academic and consultancy advice 'on both sides' of the PCT question was partially incorporated, as the Secretary of State back-tracked; backbench MPs organised around the Health Select Committee (now comprising disappointed ex-Ministers) kicked up a stink; and institutional compromises were made piecemeal, based on different and incompatible policy objectives.

For example, the government had originally wished to merge PCTs so that they could effectively commission hospital services which were increasingly organised across area networks to fulfil criteria both of quality and economy. Yet academic research on the merits of 'local commissioning' (actually conducted in the 1990s around GP fund-holding and so-called 'Total Purchasing Pilot' projects) (see for example Mays and Dixon, 1996) was now regurgitated, as part of an 'expert led' defence of local PCTs. This was useful to local 'special interests' in giving their lobbying a veneer of science. And so, given the 'political stink', the terms of debate soon shifted away from the government's original objective.

Ideologically speaking, the aim of 'patient choice' was to promote the perception that 'consumerism' could be compatible with the NHS, to head off right-wing attacks at the pass. Yet the increasing political and bureaucratic compromises between commissioning by PCTs, referrals by GPs and choice by patients, on the one hand, and between all of these and the surreptitious policy of cutting (NHS) hospital capacity to solve financial deficits (an endemic problem in 2004/5 which worsened in 2005/6), meant that neither coherent planning nor meaningful choice prevailed.

The Stages Reviewed ...

Overall then, just as a 'garbage can' approach is useful as – part of – the explanation of each strand of policy, it is also useful in explaining how the different strands are (not) reconciled, in the short term. In the long term, the story is different. Policy has to be rationalised, so that the demanding agenda confronting the welfare state in the era of globalisation is tackled. But the destabilising forces of the 'garbage can' are always threatening to undo this necessity.

A 'rational' approach to policy would lead to change as the result of evidence that objectives were not being met, on the one hand, and a plan to implement the new policy, on the other hand. In the case of the above stages, there was partial evidence that Stage 1's policy (collaboration) was not sufficient, but in reality the judgement was premature. Stage 2 (targets policed and 'performance managed' from above) may indeed have been responsible for improvements in the NHS, as even marketeers such as le Grand will concede they can be in the short term (le Grand, 2006) Indeed if Stage 4 (the new market) is found to bring benefits in terms of productivity or quality, it may well be Stage 2's mechanisms (Alvarez-Rosete et al, 2005) which are ironically responsible – as 'top down' performance management accompanies rather than yields to the market.

Part 3 of this book explores how the new policy strands introduced by each stage are forced to co-exist, in policy 'overload' – politicians are good at new initiatives but not at removing or rationalising the institutions of previous initiatives.

Cyclical waves of policy over both the 1990s and the subsequent years of New Labour have created a service in which incentives and institutions are multiple and poorly coordinated. This ironically creates the need for 'political managers' (Regional or SHA Chief Executives, in the main) to make as much sense as they can of the system and issue orders or entreaties to Trusts to comply. The watchword is 'external regulation' (in the context of devolution); the reality however is haphazard, short-termist political management of the 'market'.

The 'garbage can' has to be cleansed. But it is a tough job. Some advisers prioritise patient choice of hospitals. Others wish to rationalise and cut the acute hospital system. Some wish to do both simply because they do not understand what they are talking about. 'Payment by results' (PBR) is presented as a means of cutting bloated budgets in hospitals. But for many hospitals, being paid properly for what they do would mean more not less income, as currently – even with PBR – PCTS can't pay for the cases their GPs send to hospital, and so don't!

Some advisers want to devolve commissioning to GP practices; others want PCTs to retain responsibility. 'Managing demand' is the main rationale for stronger commissioning. Yet it might restrict choice, if patients do not want 'community alternatives' to hospital (assuming they are effective) which always sound 'politically correct' – and which respondents to consultations may choose as 'citizens' but mistrust as 'consumers'.

More generally, the tensions are between:

(1) national priorities and local choice
(2) 'scientific', evidence-based services and special lobbies; and
(3) improvement by markets ('exit') or by patient involvement to improve local services by 'voice'

The policy strands analysed in the 'stages' considered above are not however developed by reference to objectives, nor are the incentives and institutions which they create analysed as to whether they advance or retard the government's future plans. In other words, strategy is absent when policy is made, and developed 'on the hoof' as policy is implemented.

Political Institutions under New Labour

Let us consider the role of the 'backbench MP' and Parliament, on the one hand, under New Labour; and the role of the executive, on the other:

Labour MPs under New Labour

It has become a truism that, at Westminster, Parliament has lost even more power in recent years than in the 1960s and 1970s when the topic was much debated. Against this, it may be objected that, both under the Major government from 1992 to 1997 and after 2005 in New Labour's third term with a reduced majority, backbenchers and indeed the House of Lords have inflicted significant pressure and actual defeats upon the government of the day. My aim here is more limited but also different – to present a 'cultural picture' of how MPs often react to, rather than help develop, English health policy, and to suggest that the picture presented is a typical one, capable of generalisation to other policy issues.

Let me stereotype the typical backbencher under New Labour as subscribing to a 'pledgecard' approach to policy', a 'tickbox' approach to enactment (which it mistakes for implementation); a 'soundbite' approach to communication; and a sense of 'deliverables' to the constituency as 'symbolic pork' (not even real pork, US-style!) To explain:

One of the regular cries from the Labour Left in the 1960s and (especially) 1970s – the two decades of modern times, before New Labour's accession in 1997, when Labour governments predominated – was of 'betrayal' by the leadership and the Labour government. Others, such as former Minister Roy Hattersley, have been dismissive of such claims by other former Ministers such as Tony Benn (1989) arguing that, of the alleged 'broken promises', some had never been made and others had been kept (Hattersley, 1995). Ironically, after more than two terms of New Labour government, Hattersley has made a claim similar in spirit to Benn before him: that, while some promises have been 'technically' kept, they have been so trivial that the spirit if not the letter of the Labour agenda has been betrayed; that people expect an ethos from a Labour government which has been absent.

It is here that the '**pledgecard**' phenomenon comes in. New Labour's obsession pre- and post-1997 was about credibility. Some of this was about credibility with the City and international financial institutions, embodied in policies such as making the Bank of England 'autonomous', sticking to the outgoing Conservative government's published plans for public expenditure, and setting out the Chancellor's 'golden rule' for balancing public 'investment' (often actually expenditure) over the 'economic cycle'. It was also about credibility with the public, geared to ensuring that a perception of 'promises kept' helped re-election of Labour and the attainment of that historical first – (at least) two full continuous terms of office. Hence the promulgation of 'simple, easily understood' promises, embodied in the 'five promise pledgecard', which included inter alia the promise to 'cut NHS waiting lists by 100,000' (from an inherited total of over one million).

This promise was simplistic, in that waiting lists in themselves mean little. Given that waiting lists are for 'elective' rather than emergency treatment, one million people waiting a week in effect means no problem, whereas one million people waiting a year means crisis. The point here is however to point to a more general phenomenon – that the culture of policy and delivery was that of the 'shopping list' (as befits the modern voter as consumer with low attention span) rather than that of the integrated political programme.

It is important to be fair: there is no suggestion that Old Labour governments promulgated integrated programmes, still less that the Labour left in opposition brought effective practical influence to bear on behalf of its aspirations. (Consider the 1983 Labour manifesto, described by shadow cabinet member Gerald Kaufman as the 'longest suicide note in history' – although it might be argued that the whiff of suicide was more the result of incoherent compromises between the Left (Bennite), traditional 'Labourism' (as represented by the likes of John Smith), more intellectually-minded social democracy (the Crosland tradition e.g. Hattersley) and the 'unwilling monetarism' introduced by the IMF crisis of 1976, reluctantly embodied by Callaghan and Healey).

Nevertheless the **shopping list** is now a deliberate executive strategy. Arguably this has promoted a culture whereby different groups of backbenchers, of different original political orientation, respond in kind – either in agreement or with their own variant of the list. Crucially, the death of politics as ideological conflict in an era of 'global capitalist inevitability' has hastened this trend: when the left lost public ownership and economic planning and the social democrats lost Keynesian political economy, 'real Labour' backbenchers were left with localism and shopping lists. ('All politics is local", according to former US House Speaker Tip O'Neill (Farrell, 2001) 'but not as local as this, for God's sake!' might be the rider from frustrated backbenchers).

That is why it is accurate to describe Blairism as Thatcherism with a human face – 'there is no alternative' in political economy, and the task is to seek to generalise the advantages of Thatcherism to the excluded. Even health policy in the third term provides a classic example of influence by advisers whose stance is in effect, 'there's nothing wrong with bourgeois individualism – the challenge is to involve more on that basis' – hence choice as a mantra rather than a competing value.

From pledgecard to 'tickbox' – the dialogue with the electorate about accomplishments is barely about the sort of society which has been achieved but about piecemeal enactments rather than implementation (geared to social outcomes)…reminiscent of the impersonator Mike Yarwood 'doing' then-PM Harold Wilson in the 1960s and boasting, "I gave you one World Cup and two Eurovision song contests"! Every time a New Labour Minister is asked what the real aims and accomplishments are, a list rather than a vision or mission en route to realisation is generally forthcoming – which means ironically that what achievements there are (especially through the use of 'stealth taxes') are undersold, to boot. (Toynbee and Walker, 2005)

Communication too, rather than symphony, easily becomes staccato lists, informed by the soundbite; it is not too fanciful to trace this to executive documents – such as the NHS Plan of 2000 and its follow-up documents over the next couple of years – in which the verb-less sentences of the Prime Minister and the neologistic 'New Labour-speak' of Health Minister Alan Milburn shine out amongst the sections written in officialese (reflecting 'sofa government' with breathless interjection rather than coherent analysis the order of the day).

With modern Executive dominance in the form of Prime Ministerial and Chancellor's control of policy, supplemented by 'post-modern' piecemeal policy, backbench MPs find it easier to boast of 'pork' than of principles. In the US, the culture of 'pork-barrelling' in order to 'bring home the bacon' to constituencies and special interests is aided by the relative absence of ideological conflict in domestic politics between markets and planning, on the one hand, and the weakness of political parties allied to the decentralised operation of Congress. In England now, (pseudo-) localism is developing in a very different context – of strong parties deciding policy, with domestic policy resultingly centralised when one adds in the top-heavy Executive and centralist English state (despite the superficial rhetoric about local control applied to specific policy areas such as health). It is symbolic pork, not real pork, that backbenchers bring home i.e. it is spin and illusion, unlike in the US where pork has to be real or elections are lost (with less tradition of voting for the national party at district or state level even in national elections).

MPs and Health Policy – Impotence disguised as 'Symbolic Pork'-Barrelling

The above phenomenon can be illustrated from health policy. In 1997, New Labour wished to abolish GP fund-holding yet retain 'primary care' commissioning (whatever that meant, and they were genuinely unsure). This meant, at first, Primary Care Groups working as committees of the health authorities (about 100 covering England), which were 'rolled out' to become Primary Care Trusts (PCTs), at first gradually and then in a 'big bang' in 2001-2. (This mirrored the Conservatives' 1991 policy of NHS 'Self-Governing' Trusts having been voluntary at first, with a lot of meaningless 'community consultation', then mandatory; we are seeing it again with Foundation Trusts, at first to be an 'elite' wedge and now to be mandatory for hospitals at least by 2007-8.)

When PCTs were created, there was a tension between their 'commissioning'/ purchasing role and their role in providing services outside the hospital, from GP services through to community care for vulnerable groups. The latter argued for small PCTs; the former for large ones. This tension bedevilled PCTs from the start and led to the need to 're-disorganise' the NHS yet again almost straight away, but action only coming in 2005 after the election was out of the way. (See Part 3 for more detailed examination of health policy at this time, including Foundation Trusts and whether or not the 'new NHS market' allows coherent and equitable provision of services.)

The concern here however is with parliamentarians. MPs, and of course local councillors and other street-level lobbyists, generally argued for PCTs small enough to be seen as 'theirs.' (Just as there were too many small 'NHS Trusts' created between 1991 and 1993, far too many small PCTs were created by 2002.) This was however as nothing by comparison with the campaign to 'save' small PCTs in 2005-6, when the government was seeking to merge them and change their functions (See Part 3). In my home area of North Staffordshire, for example, there are five Labour MPs – two unequivocally 'Old Labour'; a former junior Minister who lost office in 2005; and two newer incumbents less easy to categorise (in other words, the 'disaffected, the dispossessed and the not-yet-disappointed' – a mixture of orientations).

PCTs are generally seen by health policy researchers in terms of whether or not they are effective in (respectively) commissioning and providing services for their populations (Mays et al, 2001). This however misses a whole dimension, just as seeing Foundation Trusts in terms of the justifications or otherwise proffered by economists and misses much of the political reality. The government too may have a clear aim for such institutions (e.g. economic efficiency and 'leanness' being the main one for Foundation Trusts) but the unintended effects are political as well as economic. Here the concern is political.

PCTs and local politics become mutually embedded. Special interests, councillors and MPs – along with Non-Executive Directors of PCTs with links to them – create a tendency (Dyson, 2003) towards 'special interest satisfaction' rather than 'population needs assessment'.

Consider, the arguments used in favour of retaining small PCTs in 2005-6, once they were threatened by *Commissioning a Patient-Led NHS* (DoH, 2005):

(1) they improve services for patients (yet in reality they often seek to lengthen their populations' waiting times to the maximum allowed by national targets, in order to save money).

(2) they 'hold the hospital to account' (yet could do so much better if merged onto a scale to give them countervailing power ......and in any case, 'holding to account' often means power without responsibility i.e. seeking to have patients treated without properly reimbursing the hospital, as under the 1990s internal market (Paton et al, 1998).

(3) they will put local people first (but this may mean that parochialism rules).

(4) they will create new services locally (but often at the expense of properly investing in services on the required scale over the wider area – hence (1) above).

(5) they 'provide what the manifesto stated' (eg 'walk-in centres'; new GP out-of-hours services...but see (4) above: in particular, they may eschew more effective options such as provision of 'out-of-hours' care by the local Ambulance Service on grounds of the 'not invented here' syndrome);

In other words, the 'pork' that local MPs bring is often 'symbolic pork'. The pledges which are ticked off and listed for constituents at election time are generally new agencies and processes – 'inputs and outputs' rather than 'outcomes'. And the 'opportunity cost' of these may mean the 'local right' to a worse service, through unnecessarily high management and service costs from retaining too many separate statutory organisations with their own sectional agendas.

This is not trivial – the 'management costs' of Shifting the Balance of Power (2001), with its plethora of PCTs and SHAs, can be estimated at £1.5 billion annually – a fact not lost on the Times' Health Editior, Nigel Hawkes (Paton, 2006b).

New Labour in government has sought 'devolution' in the NHS in order to devolve responsibility and blame rather than power – a lesson they have learned and built on from the 1990s Conservative administrations. Yet local involvement, as well as having the advantage of tying up local activists in 'administration' rather than political ferment, can resemble what happened in Disney's Fantasia when the Sorcerer left the Apprentice (Mickey Mouse) in charge...lots of little brooms came to life and started, busily and self-righteously, to help out and do the work – but without any idea of coordination or closure, leading to flood and disaster Just as the Conservatives before them found that the 'market' was a tiger which could devour its master, New Labour is (or should be) finding that its uneasy mix of market and parochialism is threatening what could be its biggest achievements – the wise spending of record sums on the NHS (see Part 3).

The Executive

Turning to the executive: the 'networks' which influence and produce health policy are indeed based in the 'core' and extended Executive (not least because the NHS is separate from local government and only tangentially linked to wider 'local governance' (Stoker (Ed), 2000). They are best conceived of as a triangle with apex at the top, composed of the Prime Minister and his office, which then widens out to include different camps of political adviser; academic advisers; 'the new civil servants' as described above, more dependent on political patronage than was Sir Humphrey in his heyday; sometime-'insider' NHS managers; and the 'new managerial elite' within the medical profession such as the clinical 'Czars' (Directors of policy for clinical services) at the Department of Health. (Since the term 'Czar' is official, we must assume that Ministers see the NHS as pre-Stalinist rather than post-Stalinist!)

There have been structural and cultural changes which have changed the nature of the 'healthcare settlement' between the state and the medical profession, as described originally by Rudolf Klein (1990) memorably in terms of the 'politics of the double bed', but with doctors now as mechanics in a garage at the beck and call of consumers rather than priests in church with humble supplicants, again to draw on Klein's metaphors. New Labour is groping its way, though its 'public service reform', towards a neo-Fordist, integrated service (see Chapter 2, above) rather than a corporatist service in which the different guilds and interests settle their differences in semi-voluntary, semi-statutory institutions. Below, at the end of Part 2, I set out briefly how the politics of the double-bed has become a struggle for space in the single bed: the political and bureaucratic executive, the major structure of the state, no longer seeks compromise with a countervailing 'structural force', the medical profession; but instead seeks to subjugate it to the corporate (but not corporatist) mission of the state – a 'unitarist' health service in pursuit of both a productive economy and a satisfied 'consuming public.'

In a nutshell, the 'new Brahmins' in health policy are the managerialists (including economists) rather than the doctors. The declining social and political power of the traditional professions (with the exception so far of the legal profession, despite the Lord Chancellor's recent reforms) is part-cause and part-consequence of a changing 'elite', composed of overlapping 'insider' networks, in health policy.

Managerialism is the glue which attempts to deliver the ambitious, often contradictory, mission for the welfare state in the era of capitalist globalization, as analysed in Part I of this book. Yet it is unstable, and also regularly undermined by 'voices off'– those helping to fill the garbage can of ideas, proposals and ideologies.

Academics and the Garbage Can – Wider Networks Influencing the Executive?

A concluding word in this section is reserved for academic advisors and policy analysts influencing the Executive. There are 'insider' series of networks and the 'outsider' policy communities (Marsh, 1998). Straddling the two are the prominent 'media academics' who have commented on, and advised on, NHS policy over the last twenty years; and also the 'primary care' advocates, including the Institute for Public Policy Research (IPPR), and other metropolitan 'think tanks'.

Regarding the former, we can identify the technocrat, who bemoans the irrational and malign influence of politics upon the agenda of evidence-based effectiveness and formalised utility-measurement. There is also the pragmatist, always 'on board' but leaning just-and-no-more to the port-side of the agenda of the day. Then there is the ideologist in recent years, combining a love of markets with a left-of-centre desire to help the worse-off. The latter has become a 'primary care commissioning' industry, dusting off its 1990s research aimed at advising the Conservatives how best to organise GP and local purchasing, as Labour moves to Practice-Based Commissioning (Smith et al, 2005). From the 1980s to the present day, different combinations of academic advice have reflected the ethos of the day, with markets to the fore now. All the same, the inputs are plural rather than chronological or rational.

What all share is a mode of analysis which takes health reform proposals from (and to) government at 'face value.' When they are disappointed, they see accident rather than design. They do not perceive their own influence as reflective of the garbage can, but as sensible! They all have a tendency to meet politics with analysis, as if one can persuade the other. It might be said that only a conspiracy theorist would be otherwise. Yet there is a middle way between being ingenuous and seeing conspiracy: that is to explore the political origins of policy as well as its internal analytics, and to have a 'nose' for the political management of policy implementation. Much health policy 'insider' advice falls foul of what economists call 'the problem of the second best': a solution is only optimal under certain conditions; and when these do not pertain, the solution may be worse than alternatives.

The largely untold story in health policy since 1991 concerns the pitfalls (Pressman and Wildavsky, 1973) of implementation. The politics of health reform has been told in 'comparative statics', or how different reform proposals originated from different political stables in different countries. But the story of how aims are subverted has only been told summarily (i.e. it happened) or anecdotally. The main reasons for subversion lie in: the tacit political agenda behind reforms as opposed to the justifying theory; the need to render different policy strands compatible with each other and with changing political streams; and unintended consequences flowing from the manner in which the 'analytics' of reform interact with the 'political' management of reforms.

Reviewing the Factors Influencing Public Policy

At the beginning of Part 2, I outlined the key factors used to explain public policy. Summarising heroically, these are: political economy; political structure; power; and ideas. Jumping from the sublime to the ridiculous, the million-dollar question for New Labour's health policy has been how to reconcile loose 'ideas' from the garbage can of policy initiatives, with the increasingly tight corset of political economy. In other words, in terms of the continuum (or hierarchy) of factors explaining policy, how is the anarchy produced at one end – 'incoherent' ideas and incoherent combinations of ideas – reconciled with the key factor at the other end of the continuum – political economy? There is both a theoretical challenge – which explanatory factors are salient, or come to dominate? – and a practical challenge – who or what (if anything) rationalises the mess?

I have already suggested that the practical challenge is attempted by 'meso level' political managers. In the NHS, to be concrete, these are the Strategic Health Authority Chief Executives. They do not seek to rationalise the system because they have read academic text books on 'meso level rationalisation'. Nor do they do so because they are altruists (which they may or may not be). They do so because they are held accountable by the political Executive for 'noise' on 'their patch', which very often stems from the incoherent policy mix promulgated by those very politicians who comprise the political Executive. Thus they have a 'love-hate' relationship with their (political) masters, like all dependent denizens: they secretly despise their amateurism yet advance their careers by praising their agenda and seeking to minimise the noise. Part 3 explores the prospects – in the NHS of 2006 and beyond – of this being done sustainably.

Regarding the theoretical challenge: we can detect how the disparate policy initiatives from the garbage-can are combined over time (whether or not they are reconciled in terms of establishing policy coherence). This is where the intermediate factors which explain policy are useful.

Political Economy	Political Structure	(Culture)	Power	'Garbage Can' Ideas
LONG TERM FACTORS	INTERMEDIATE FACTORS			SHORT TERM FACTORS

Figure 4.1 Aggregate Factors Explaining Public Policy

This theoretical challenge is at a middle level of theory as opposed to 'grand theory' of a universal sort: that is, conclusions must be dependent upon the 'biases', observed empirically, engendered in individual countries and settings by intermediate factors such as political structure and the configuration of power.

In New Labour's England of the early 21st Century, we can detect a mobilisation of bias (Schattschneider, 1960) based on: (1) how **political structure** affects policy's emergence and implementation; (2) how political economy's dictates, or perceived dictates, affect ideas (or political culture); and (3) how political power is intertwined with economic power.

We can analyse the 'stages' of policy reviewed above (as explained using the concept of the garbage-can) to determine firstly what the recurring themes are, if any; and, secondly, how political structures influence the implementation and 'maintenance of policy over time. The first part of this is briefly done in Part 3 below. Meanwhile, some pointers are provided below regarding the second part.

Regarding (1), above: political structure creates a bias to centralism (the 'Westminster model') which creates a paradox for policy initiatives which are based on: devolution or decentralization; (re)introducing a market into public services; or both. For the reality is a growing rhetoric of markets and localism yet ever greater centralization. In a nutshell, the political culture of hierarchical control (semi humorously but persistently referred to as 'Stalinism' in the NHS) tends to override the analytical coherence (if such there be) of policy reforms based on economic theory. In concrete language , the tidy proposals from Prime Ministerial advisors such as Stevens (2006) and Le Grand (2003) based on rudimentary economic theory become something very different in practice. The charge of 'Stalinism' is not just an exaggerated means of pointing to top down control in organisational terms: it provides a pointer to an organizational culture, politically – derived, which encourages 'apparatchik' behaviour.

Such behaviour is (in the vernacular) part of the 'kiss up, kick down' culture, whereby personnel at higher tiers in the hierarchy (whether formal or disjointed) seek to devolve both responsibility and blame instead of collaborating on strategy to solve problems – and do so in order to 'report up' about the (non-) performance of subordinate tiers.

Thus a centralist structure may be accompanied by an apparatchik culture. This is not necessary, but regrettably has evolved thus during 'New Labour's stewardship of the NHS. It has of course occurred in direct proportion to Ministers' desperation to salvage their reputations, and NHS meso-level executives' desperation to please them in pursuit of job security, as NHS resources have grown substantially yet diminished in potential benefit as a result of 'policy overload' and confusion.

Ironically this threatens the very purpose which creates the culture in the first place – salvaging a state-funded NHS. Cultural destabilisation or degeneration is, in the long run, much more pernicious than 'x – inefficiency'. The latter can in any case be tackled in a different way – through regionally-organised state-funded services which integrate care (see Part 3). But New Labour has suffered from the same pathology in health policy as more generally: it has failed to build on and boast of its potential social-democratic achievements because it wants to emphasise its market credentials (Toynbee and Walker, 2005).

The paradox is that the advocacy of 'markets' in the NHS has abolished legitimate regional planning; ironically centralized political control as a result; and destabilised the whole NHS. The more Alan Milburn preached a renunciation of central control, the more he created new central mechanisms to control his 'de-Stalinization'. This is not 'constructive discomfort' (the phrase attributed to his former adviser Simon Stevens), but destructive masochism.

The other effect of a centralized political structure is seen when we add in 'New Labour's' 'post-modern' state – different central policies are administered down different 'silos' from centre to periphery (ie the various local NHSs). Thus 'patient choice' (the new market) is not integrated with other policies, but is a central initiative administered as if in a colonial state. In particular, it has to co-exist with 'commisioner contracting', centrally designed from a rival 'silo' (the old market). This means that, in fact, hospital trusts cannot maximise their income by maximising patient-care – the latter is controlled by limitations on contracts (as in the 1990s internal market). Additionally central targets, directly enforced through the Strategic Health Authorities and/or Monitor (see Part 3), comprise another 'silo policy' as does integrated care through collaboration in local health economies.

Analytically, it is a mess. Politically, it is both expensive and conducive to 'management by panic', whereby single issues or 'crises' dominate for short periods of time, and are addressed one-by-one. This phenomenon reached its apotheosis in 2005-6, as 'activity and targets' (pre-general election of 2005) yielded to 'finance' post-election, with each (equally, in turn) the subject of urgent directives from above.

The fact that these directives were not part of an overall strategy, except at the level of rhetoric about 'reform', was encouraged by the combination of political structure and political culture.

Turning to political economy's dictates ((2) above), 'the market' has come even more to the fore in NHS policy in the 2000s than in the early 1990s (after the brief hiatus during which New Labour 'abolished the internal market', in 1997-2000). This is policy by osmosis rather than rationality: in global political economy, the market rules (therefore, it is implied, the NHS can't be exempt.) In terms of the NHS having to live in the wider world of labour supply, 'low tax' and investment in the economy this is true. But in terms of the NHS's internal organisation, it is a non-sequitur.

Nevertheless, the cultural effect of political economy – what might be termed, the recurring idea – has meant that other (and subsequent) ideas and initiatives from the garbage can are increasingly organised within the market framework. This explains the paradox of why the 'New Labour NHS market' (administered by Blairites with former left-wing pedigrees) is more radical than the Conservatives' version. It is a question of both (political) timing and the continuing mobilisation of political bias – not a question of the rationality of the idea. The Thatcher market did some of the demolition work on the 'old culture', making it easier for Blair. The fact that, within the NHS, there was much world-weariness regarding 'history repeating itself' (as farce rather than tragedy) did not matter politically: such views were expressed below the level of 'high politics'(Klein, 2002).

Regarding (3) above – the intertwining of political power and economic power – the apparatus of the state, and particularly the executive, has increasingly been infused by representatives of private interests. This is witnessed within the

Treasury and the Department of Health, in terms of both key advisers and the decision-making machinery around policies such as the PFI (Paton, 2006a). As a result, rationalisation of disparate initiatives is, again, inevitably within a market framework. This framework is not, however, one which enables local choice as to public/private deals. It is a framework to enforce centrally-imposed 'marketisation' and privatisation of provision – as with, respectively, PFIs (Pollock, 2004) and use of the independent sector for treatment.

Thus, overall, the 'garbage can's' initiatives are shaped by power: one has to investigate in whose backyard the garbage can is situated.

And the Political Result?

Is it possible that, on health, New Labour will be judged to have snatched defeat from the jaws of victory? That is, will its aim of modernising and therefore preserving state-funded healthcare have backfired, because policy confusion and 'overload' undermined the NHS both economically and politically?

There is certainly a large 'management overhead cost' to New Labour's four conflicting policy strands – and in particular the 'costs of commissioning' – which I have estimated as at least three times the NHS national deficit in England for 2006 (Paton, 2006b). When one adds to this the direct costs of pay awards, target achievement and central financing of the private sector, the conclusion emerges that – with the resources provided – New Labour could have provided much more healthcare than they did up to 2006, even before 'reform'. The questions for further 'reform' are then: it is intrinsically necessary, or is it rendered necessary by the pressure put upon providers (hospitals in particular) by the wasting of resources elsewhere; and, if necessary, should it emphasise market relations within the NHS or greater collaborative integration?

In Part 2, I have sought to emphasise that how politics affects the policies which provide answers to such questions is seriously under-explored in practice.

Part 3 examines dominant ideas, which have come to dominate different stages of reform and re-organisation of the NHS. That is, it continues with the theme of a 'mobilisation of bias' in ongoing reform (for political and organisational reasons) rather than a reform agenda which is rationally based upon coherent goals and evidence as to how best to achieve these.

The ultimate question for the NHS is: can it survive politically and organisationally; or has the garbage-can left a smell which cannot be eradicated? If the latter, then replacement of the NHS by a pluralistic, private-dominated system will have been hastened by cock-up rather than conspiracy (Paton, 2001). It will have been occasioned by a New Labour own goal rather than an effective strike from the NHS's opponents.

Chapter 5

Implementation: Power, Political Structure, Health Policy and the 'New Regulation'

Paradigms of Policy

Some of the conventional literature on public policy is rather stale and tautologous – and 'technical' rather than political. Many textbooks essentially argue that, when all the necessary conditions for making policy effective exist together, policy will be made. But a more significant problem is that, when it comes to innovative and seminal work, it appears in different 'schools' which do not have a common frame of reference. For example, those writers who start with the distribution of power in society and government (leading to the great political sociology debates of the 1960s and 1970s, ranging from Dahl (1980) through Bachrach and Baratz (1970) to Crenson (1971) and Lukes (1974), are not 'compared and contrasted' with the pragmatic institutionalism of the likes of Allison (1971) writing at the same time. Allison devised three models of the government machine – respectively: rationality, bureaucracy and political bargaining.

It is sometimes implied (Dunleavy and O'Leary, 1982) that Allison's three models are all basically pluralist. But they are not, for they are not based on an analysis of social power. They are models of the central government machine, which may or may not apply to the wider distribution of social power; may or may not apply outside the USA; may or may not apply to domestic as opposed to foreign (and particularly security) policy; and which, specifically regarding Allison's Model 1, may or may not equate 'rationality' with consensus established on the basis of pluralism, as opposed to rationality actually being the voice of the dominant faction in decision-making.

That indeed is the difference between studies of (political) executive decision-making, on the one hand, and the empirical studies of power, on the other: the former are about decisions *within* a policy framework, and the latter are about the *making* of policy (and who benefits as well as who rules). But political science, in its search for typologies and comparisons, has lost sight of the obvious.

The assumption of 'rationality as public interest' in policy decisions is that the state is autonomous of class or partial interest. An alternative is that 'rationality' is the orthodoxy of a ruling class, an elite or a bureaucracy with its own interest which is 'autonomous' of other elites but separate from the public interest. This leads us to another fork in the road in analysing policy. How do we understand how different political institutions in different countries (or even, to modernize the debate, in different multi-national organizations) produce different results, or at least different ways of configuring power?

Another schism in analysis, as observed above, fails to distinguish between rationality and maximisation (the link to the influence of neo-classical economics upon political science.) Rationality is the tailoring of means to ends on the basis of 'agreed ends', whatever that means, but maximisation is what it says. And is the latter 'consensual maximisation' on behalf of the public interest, or is it different interests all seeking to maximise their benefit in terms of their sectional aims…in which case, what rules and structures mediate the result? Does a pluralist plethora of interests engaged in maximisation produce (by compromise and/or log-rolling) an incrementalism in policy output? Much in U.S. domestic policy, at least, would suggest so (Paton, 1990).

A key concern is the interplay between power, political structure and policy-making. 'Power' includes the area described in Part 1 as political economy. In particular, this may shed light on whether the design and operation of policy is geared 'internally' or 'externally': is health policy, for example, designed with the health sector in mind or with wider economic factors in mind? A good example of the latter in the NHS is the Private Finance Initiative, created by the Conservatives in 1990 and extended by New Labour. This uses private capital to build 'public' hospitals, with the NHS paying back the capital investment by private consortia in the form of annual 'revenue' payments over thirty years or more. This policy is mostly about removing capital investment from government accounts, to reduce the 'public sector borrowing requirement'; and is certainly not designed with the specific needs of the health sector in mind. Transfer of powers within NHS decision-making, to private banks and corporations, is mirrored by the wider location of power over public policy within 'central networks' which bring together government, commercial and financial interests. The Treasury (Capital Investment Branch), central units in other government departments (eg the Department of Health's Private Finance Unit), 'PFI advisers' from the consultancy and banking world and the 'elite' consortia bidding for PFI contracts comprise a private/public 'sub-government'.

More widely, the analysis of Part 1 showed how the 'demands' of political economy may influence domestic and social policy, as with health. This is a form of power – quasi-functionalist, in that it is 'the system' which causes it. It is important to demonstrate who wields – or allows – this power, however; otherwise there is a lapse into structural-functionalism which underplays the role of human agency. The latter is always possible: it is just that the collective, international nature of such in the era of global capitalism is daunting. In the case of the analysis in Part 1 above, the empirical, 'instrumental' power is held 'positively' by government but (more significantly) 'negatively' by international financial institutions, international organisations such as the WTO and the EU and the domestic economic elite (with the media playing an important role), all of which would quickly mobilise against government were it to seek to change the prevailing political economy.

When analysing power, therefore, it is important to distinguish between 'external power' which affects a policy area or issue such as health but which is not exerted with health as the primary consideration, on the one hand, and 'internal power' exerted within the health arena, on the other hand.

The latter may be exerted during either the policy-making phase or the implementation phase. It is important not to be too theological in making this distinction (after all, the 'policy process' is continual and even circular) but the distinction holds some heuristic value. For example, in the US, where domestic policy with welfare, distributionist or redistributionist implications (Lowi, 1964; Paton, 1990) usually requires either 'log-rolling' or compromise to bring the representatives of different interests together in Congress, the relevant actors (especially those powerful groups threatened by the proposal) usually have significant input during the policy-making phase. If this is so, there may be less opposition during the implementation phase (there is less to oppose!) – although one should not underestimate the complexity inherent in implementing social reform in a federal system when Oakland is a long way from Washington DC (Pressman and Widavsky, *op.cit*) and where the political culture militates against implementation by 'command and control.'

In the UK, the centralised government structure means that it is possible for a strong governing party to pass legislation on the basis of 'majority rule' or 'strongest wins.' It should be admitted that today, given the prevailing political economy and political culture which it promulgates, this is less likely – especially if the 'sub-government' elites are active behind the scenes. But it can still occur. If it does, it may offend powerful groups who have not been consulted or involved in design or compromise. It is therefore during the implementation phase that conflict and/or compromise may occur.

Implementation, Social Power and State Control

We can see an example of this with the 'NHS Plan' of 2000, which set out a framework for (in the government's words) "investment and reform" for the NHS. Ironically, it was not meant to be like that: the government's intention was to create a 'big tent', counting in all the major 'health interests' in the creation of the NHS Plan. Testimony to this is provided by the signatures of many key players on the NHS Plan document – ranging from Presidents of medical Royal Colleges, through the British Medical Association, the Royal College of Nursing, representatives of NHS Boards, NHS management (and the workforce) and representatives of patients and citizens' organisations. The problem is that the 'consultation' was a post-modern pick-and-mix, with the real issues reserved for the implementation phase. What looked like a wonderful rainbow coalition of unlikely bedfellows soon began to fray at the edges –

most notably when the section of the Plan dealing with 'professions' led to proposed new contracts for doctors. These sought to increase accountability of consultants to NHS Trusts in return for more money for those doctors who committed themselves more substantially to the NHS than the previous contract stipulated. The President of the Royal College of Surgeons was soon in hot water with many of his members for having blithely signed the Plan! On resigning, the Department of Health's Director of Human Resources blamed Ministers for having abused the consensual goodwill of 2000 (Foster, 2006).

The wider issue is the power of the medical profession, which is slowly declining but still significant in the eyes of many health policy commentators who have seen this as 'the' pivotal power issue in healthcare. Doctors are characterised as 'the power elite.' Yet this is misleading, in the absence of clarification. They may be at or near the top of a hierarchy internal to healthcare. Yet (mostly) publicly-employed doctors, however well-remunerated or otherwise, are not part of the 'external' power elite which sets the agenda for health policy and the NHS, as analysed in Part 1 above.

They are not an elite in terms of their relation to political economy in general and capital in particular. In this context, NHS doctors are the 'new proletariat', (albeit the best-paid bunch of exploited workers!) – no longer a self-governing guild based on self-regulated 'craft work' but becoming (the government hopes) part of the neo-Fordist machine described in Part 1 above. The public NHS is the most cost-effective means of organising investment in health, and doctors are employees whose surplus value is extracted, where possible, to increase surplus value economy-wide, through healthier workers being more profitable. (Paton, 2001)

This 'macro' purpose for the NHS is an 'ideal type' of course, used to exaggerate a point in order to make it. It implies a 'rational' strategy on the part of government as if there were a 'unitarist' mission for the NHS (i.e. all key players pulling in the same direction). Internally, it may be a different story. Doctors may either resist the mission incrementally, using their power as 'street level bureaucrats' to make local priorities, including whom they treat how, which are different from the government's plan (or Plan). Alternatively they may resist more radically. That is where 'NHS reform' comes in: it is not based on politicians reading elegant economics textbooks' homilies about markets but primarily about 'dividing and ruling' within the medical profession (as true with New Labour reform in the 2000s as with Conservative reform in the 1990s).

'Who wins' in the long run is crucial for the future of the NHS. The state seeks to ensure adequate implementation by the medical (and other) professions of what it sees as the agenda required to ensure the economic functionality and political legitimacy of the NHS. If this does not happen, both private employers and the 'post-Fordist' right-of-centre electoral coalition may eventually give up on the NHS.

In the past, the unwritten concordat between the medical profession and the state traded off autonomy for doctors at the 'meso' level (Moran, 1999) for compliance with state-determined levels of funding for the NHS in general and the doctors' salary bill and education/training budgets, in particular. NHS funding and internal politics were kept below the 'radar screen', out of 'high politics.' This was tenable in the age of the 'Keynesian national welfare state' (Jessop, 2002) when: international competition and dependence on mobile capital was less; medical possibilities (and therefore budgetary pressures) were less; and consumerism and 'active citizenship' made many fewer demands upon the service. It is less tenable today.

In essence, the 'low morale' of the medical profession today stems from anomie, an uncertainty as to their position and indeed as to what it might be or should be. Yes, there are greedy doctors who are simply annoyed that their snouts are being removed from the trough, or even that their feeding at the trough is being monitored. But they are a small minority. At the other extreme, there are idealists who either can be trusted to 'regulate themselves' or think they can. But in between, there are the masses of hospital doctors who feel the pressure of both 'government targets' and what they see as 'half-baked reforms', on the one hand, and GPs with less 'out-of-hours' work than even eminent consultant Professors, on the other hand.

The 'two worlds' of policy do not meet. On the one hand, there is the politicians' world of targets and initiatives to keep the momentum, to ensure that demanding patients and their families do not give bad publicity to the NHS as a result of long waits, 'cancelled operations' or unresolved complaints. On the other hand, there is the clinical world, often puzzled as to why politicians cannot see the 'perverse outcomes' from targets and funding regimes. There are many such outcomes: for example, 'maximum waiting times' mean that trivial cases may be prioritised over more serious cases. Postponement of operations, for which the patient had already been given a date, to the next financial year were a feature of 2005-6, given hospital deficits, for patients waiting for only a few days less than others, who were seen immediately – on the grounds that they would have 'breached' targets if held over. At clinical 'street level' this seems absurd.

The question for politicians is whether the 'negatives' for patients and doctors from the 'target regime' or equivalent are outweighed by the 'positive' of more productivity overall in the search for an NHS which is economically sustainable as a 'socialist island in a capitalist world'. The danger is that the ethos of a major service cannot be insulated from its external environment, not least when that environment is the source of its financing and employment and a major influence on what (and how) it must provide.

In this environment – rather than keeping its 'eye on the ball' of its ambitious mission to provide an NHS which aided the economy, kept the middle-classes quiet and tackled some health inequalities (all of which required a stable strategy) – New Labour seemed to panic in the headlights, seeing 'permanent revolution' as the means of keeping the NHS on its toes. To quote Hyman (2005) again, "our approach to political strategy had been based on three things: momentum, conflict and novelty, whereas the frontline requires empowerment, partnership and consistency" (p.384).

And so we are back to the garbage can, albeit in the context of the state's need for a 'rational strategy' and (admittedly often implicit) search for one; only this time, the garbage can pouring its contents into implementation rather than policy design.

Problems of Implementation

The 'garbage can' recycles initiatives from politicians, solutions from partisans and analyses from academics. Policy initiatives come from politicians in response to politicians' problems, politicians' perception and interpretation of problems and the filtering of problems and perceptions by political advisers, interests and the media. This is a different world from the purer one inhabited by analysts and academics. Politicians have agendas e.g. re-election as a result of meeting targets they have set for themselves and (sometimes) ideological objectives. Partisan thinkers and 'think-tanks' have 'solutions in search of problems' (e.g. 'markets, decentralisation and purchaser/provider splits, in healthcare, which became the new orthodoxy without an evidence-base).

Purer analysts have evidence and (occasionally) solutions in response to the analysis of problems, but often problems analysed within a purely empiricist framework. For example, well-meaning analysts may perceive New Labour's health policy to have failed because new moneys have not been used 'cost-effectively'. Yet such diagnoses are often as hasty and premature as politicians' policies – and based on a failure to define the whole picture. For example, 'total numbers of surgical operations conducted in one year' is fairly meaningless, yet in 2003 the King's Fund (of London) noted a decline in this total – with the government's policy of 'investment and reform' thereby allegedly on the ropes. Yet productivity may still have increased, if one adjusted for quality, increased complexity of cases on waiting lists, increased use of resources by emergencies, and supply-side bottlenecks caused by EU working-time directives. In 2005, the O.E.C.D. in Paris and both the Office of National Statistics (ONS) and the Reform 'think tank', in London, pointed to declining NHS productivity. Yet the picture presented was partial. Judgement on the basis of naïve numbers over inappropriate timeframes is at the end of the day as 'partial' as screaming headlines by tabloid newspapers.

A major problem for implementation stems from these 'different worlds'. Politicians, advocates of solutions to problems and those responsible for implementation may have different perceptions as well as different values. As a result, who 'wins' in the implementation process depends upon the distribution of power in both policy-making and implementation. Politicians may or may not be able to rely upon 'command and control', steering and other approaches. Such factors will themselves depend upon political structure (e.g. can central direction overcome federalism or the institutional power of different professions and interests).

Another problem for implementation is that politicians may allow clashing incentive systems, each based on different policy strands, to lead to organisational gridlock and even demoralisation. The NHS since 1997 is a case in point. The combination of different strands is not rational. One cannot have a technical answer to a non-technical problem.

Next, policy per se may be non-rational (in the sense of coherent ends translated into coherent initiatives capable of step-wise or integrated achievement through coherent means.) For example, health policy is media- and public-driven, with the symbiosis of media-driven public opinion and public-driven media opinion producing a mix of insight and populism. For example, shorter waiting times matter, as does minimising cancelled operations; so does good quality emergency care ('no trolley waits'). Higher-level performance indicators in the NHS also measure things (imperfectly) which matter, ranging from overall health outcomes, through outcomes of operations, through staff satisfaction, through patients satisfaction and so on. But the way these are combined into targets and policed may be haphazard and fragmented, or at least contested.

If so, the only way to create a consensus is to work at 'undistorted communication' involving Ministers and elected representatives, professionals, managers and public representatives. One must distinguish between unanimity, consensus, coherent compromise and incoherent compromise. Even if unanimity at the level of 'deepest values' is possible (Paton, 1992b), different weight may be given to different, shared values (Gray, 1995). What is more, apparent 'values' involving policy choices, even if amenable to change as a result of evidence, may be essentially contested. As a result,' day to day' policy is likely to require either consensus or compromise.

Consensus is a difficult option, and political systems with strong executives and strong Premiers within them are likely to operate as 'the fastest law in the West' (Hill, 1997), as in the UK and New Zealand. In New Zealand health reform has occurred in some respects in similar fashion to that in the UK – market reforms with a 'big bang' then reversal (Paton et al, 2000). Even where consensus is achieved it may be superficial (e.g. the NHS Plan in 2000 in England) or compromise masquerading as consensus – yet incomplete compromise, suggesting 'trouble ahead'. Furthermore 'instant reaction', by media and public, militate strongly against 'undistorted communication' and 'deliberative democracy' in pursuit of consensus. Governments and oppositions will see political opportunities from creating or encouraging such reaction.

Compromise may be either coherent or incoherent, as regards the internal analytics of policy. Political systems based on compromise (e.g. the US, in domestic policy) may produce policy which can then be implemented with less subversion. Yet the price of this may be policy 'fragments' which are piecemeal, and *in toto* less effective or radical (Paton, 1990). In other words, success in implementation is the result of failure in policy itself – hardly a type of success to treasure. For example, US federal health policy since the 1970s, covering both the (end of the) 'liberal' period and the conservative ascendancy from 1980 onwards (Clinton notwithstanding), has been fragmented and unsuccessful in its own terms, although many fragments have been implemented.

One can also look at how policy is assembled in the US. During the 'Fordist' era of the industrial welfare state, (which the US never quite reached politically although it led economically) one of the reasons that the US was a policy 'laggard' (Moran, 1999) was that its political structure militated against the coherent creation of national welfare programmes. In the US, even during 'left of centre' times, policy still had to be assembled piecemeal for each client group – reflecting the conventional political *modus operandi* and the incentives created for behaviour within the political system. Only exceptional 'crisis' blasted a way around this.

As a result, there was a mobilisation of bias away from a welfare state which was comprehensive and universal yet also affordable (Paton, 1990). During the 'right of centre' era which has followed policy has remained piecemeal – and indeed this has protected some programmes for the less well-off (Farrell, 2001). This is because Congressional 'log-rolling' and other features of the system have prevented a dismantling of the progressive settlement. The Reagan strategy, for example – after the economic slump which led to Democrat gains in Congress in the mid-term elections of 1982 – was a 'reverse-Keynesianism' which combined 'pork-barrel' programmes for the better-off and deficit financing, 'The hogs were really feeding', said David Stockman, Reagan's disillusioned ex-Budget Director (Stockman, 1986). To the detriment of President Bush Senior, Reagan's successor, it was the Federal Reserve Bank which eventually stopped the largesse.

Another problem in implementation concerns 'policy learning' and 'policy transfer', especially in the age of global capitalism when policies may be copied internationally – either because there are structural constraints upon the nature and shape of welfare or because there is 'faddism', fashion and copy-catting in policy. The fact that political scientists and practitioners generally live in separate worlds leads to a failure to distinguish between: real transfer of policy, and implementation; apparent transfer and implementation of policy, but of what is actually a very different policy; and, adoption of policy rhetoric due to global convergence in political economy, yet 'pick and mix' implementation. The need to distinguish among the above applies when examining how different countries 'implement differently' within a seemingly common framework of policy as in the European Union, for example (Paton et al, 2001) – and also when considering global trends. A recent international trend with great influence upon the English NHS, has been the move to 'privatisation accompanied by external regulation' as an alternative to publicly – planned and government-controlled services. New Labour in particular has followed this trend, as exemplified by Tony Blair's 'Singapore speech' shortly before taking office (Blair, 1996). The following pages consider this both as a policy per se and as a means of implementing health policy and strategy.

Regulation as Poor Implementation?

A good example of both faddism and the effect of international political economy – including policies imposed through international agencies and through the obligations of membership of international political organisations such as the European Union (EU) – is the so-called 'new regulation' in healthcare (Saltman, Busse and Mossialos (Eds.), 2002). State healthcare systems in Europe (including the Central and Eastern European countries) have been fragmented in the name of competition and market forces; and 'social insurance' systems have adopted 'managed competition' (Paton *et al*, 2000). These reforms run the risk of missing wider insights from political science, such as those offered to a European context by Lowi's (1964) consideration of redistribution, distribution, and regulation. The 'regulatory state' may be a symptom of political failure in social policy, rather than a role model to be copied.

When one considers the regulatory role of the EU through both executive and judicial means, the negative effects of replacing direct control with an 'independent regulator' can be seen. These include: detachment from policy by the latter; lack of sympathy by the latter for wider policy objectives (ie. a tendency to obey the 'letter' but not the 'spirit' of policy); and (crucially), a piecemeal or 'single case' approach. This is inevitable with a quasi-judicial function but commonly destructive of coordinated policy.

The cornerstone of New Labour's English health reforms is the creation of 'the new regulatory state', sometimes summed up as the New Governance (Scrivens, 2005). Yet in practice, command-and-control by the state is retained, although the rhetoric is of control without command. That is, 'controls assurance' or at least assurance, as to central or universal standards (or definitions of quality) is combined with devolution in pursuit of innovation. The danger however is that the political disadvantages of both command and control are retained while the advantages are abandoned.

Let us ask: what type of regulation; for what purpose; in what context?

Regulation may be promelgated in order to **develop** competitive markets – either in former state services e.g. NHSs or in 'guild' systems which have been uncompetitive e.g. Bismarckian health systems (Paton et al, 2000). Alternatively it may be designed to restrict competitive markets for social and political reasons. 'Regulation' may of course be developed for a separate purpose, without privatisation or marketisation, in an attempt to obtain the alleged benefits of independent regulation for state systems in pursuit of specific standards. The question then is how the state (if it is prepared to do so at all) shares power with the regulator e.g. in setting priorities for the health system, and then priorities and targets for regulation. The latter will impact on the former, for example by exposing underfunding as a source of poor quality (either of services of workforce conditions). Market enthusiasts may say 'the state will always crowd out the regulator'. But this can happen in any system, unless there is an independent judicial role for the regulator based on a political settlement which includes healthcare and social rights . The good side of the EU in this regard is its 'social aspirations' i.e. the European social model. The bad side is its chosen instrument, of the single market and pro-competition (Paton et al, 2001) enforced through judicial regulation which fails to see the big picture.

A key aspect of regulation is whether it is conducted by an agency external or internal to the management of the services being regulated (in the case of public services, the state, or a delegated, 'deconcentrated', decentralized or devolved variant thereof.) Indeed Day and Klein (1987) comment, plausibly, that if it is not external, it may be better not to consider it regulation (presumably being performance management instead) Let us consider some aspects of this.

The 'external regulator' is to be found in the UK in recent years in the privatised utilities and enterprises formerly in public ownership. The first question is whether it is competition, oligopoly or 'natural monopoly' which is being regulated. If it is the last of these the question should be asked, why? Are there advantages to privatisation which outweigh loss of control (not least in pursuit of social objectives or the 'public interest'), other than: obedience to external powers (e.g. the WTO or EU); getting investment 'off the government balance sheet' (even if it is more expensive to pay back in the long run); or creating the reality or appearance of a regime friendly to global capitalism. Most privatisations are 'political', and advanced for these reasons.

Consider also whether or not the 'external regulator' is as pure a specimen as generally thought. In the UK, the Bank of England's post-1997 freedom to set interest rates seems radical. Yet government sets the target (inflation), …and could even (were the orthodoxy of the age not so hostile) manage the economy though direct interaction in prices and incomes, leaving the Bank to make a technical decision. In other words, the new power is actually a technical responsibility, not a right to 'make strategy.' It is a means by which New Labour can say: 'we're not Old Labour; we're pro-capitalist; we can be trusted not to interfere'. In other words, the point is to reassure markets. In health, that particular need is not there, unless in terms of reassuring the tax payer that standards are adequate.

In health, the three key quasi- independent 'regulators' (actually meaning state bodies 'de-concentrated' from central government) since 1997 are: the National Institute for Clinical Excellence (NICE); the Healthcare Commission (formerly the Commission for Healthcare Audit and Inspection (CHAI) itself formerly the Commission for Health Improvement (CHI); and Monitor, the body created to regulate Foundation Trusts in the NHS. The first recommends whether or not drugs and technologies should be provided on the NHS. But it does not make comparative decisions within a total resource envelope. The second has seen its powers extended incrementally. It rates hospitals and other providers, in line with government-set standards and targets. That is, it is an inspector rather than a regulator – if one draws a distinction between regulating, inspecting and enforcing/managing performance. But it does not give a view as to trade-offs between quality and other system priorities. The third, Monitor, is the 'external regulator' for (hospital) Foundation Trusts (see Part 3). Its actual behaviour 'behind the scenes' is geared to ensuring the financial solvency not just of the new Foundation Trusts, but of the whole NHS. This is partly because all hospital Trusts are allegedly to become Foundations; but also because New Labour has created a 'new market' without remotely considering how it is to be regulated, let alone managed, *overall*. Thus Monitor is de facto filling a hole, which it is equipped neither theoretically nor practically to fill. Monitor is a one-club golfer ('remove the deficit') when NHS financial solvency and coherence of services requires many clubs. The financial viability of hospital Trusts depends on their contracts with their commissioners (purchasers) ie Primary Care Trusts (PCTs) and (now) GP practices (as GP fund-holding is re-invented in the form of Practice-Based Commissioning). Monitor is pulled into managing the whole health economy, rather than simply 'regulating' the market generally and criteria for individual Trust viability.

Yet Monitor – although forced to be a 'system manager' rather than (just) 'market regulator' – acts with the culture of the latter in that it views Trusts and their localities in isolation. Furthermore, rather than its economic 'regulation' being rendered compatible with the Healthcare Commission's 'capacity standards and quality' regulation, the two organisations jostle for power. More confusing still, PCTs have been given the responsibility of setting standards, post 2006. This leads to a conflict of interest, or 'passing the buck' to hospitals, or both. For if higher standards are not affordable by hospitals, PCTs may still impose them (thereby passing the buck) or alternatively (if the Healthcare Commission inspects whole health economies including PCTs) may deliberately keep standards lower so that they are achievable (thereby demonstrating a conflict of interest).

Overall, the moral is that an 'economic' rationale for a 'regulated market' may be politically naïve as well as economically naïve. 'External regulators' may be pulled into system management on behalf of the state. The functions have not changed qualitatively: it is just that the government wants to play symbolic tricks concerning the role of the state.

In healthcare, therefore, a key question should be: what are the purposes of (and strategy for) external regulation? Is it: to regulate market structure e.g. degree of competition, including factors such as degree of cooperation between providers or location of providers, with social objectives in mind; to regulate price; to regulate access; to regulate quality; or all of these? How are piecemeal external regulators to be combined without burden (Hood et al, 1999)?

Simply to assume that regulation is about making markets more perfect (for 'technical efficiency') and that other objectives are merely a 'social residue' to be dealt with separately, shows how far the New Right or neo-liberal ideology has penetrated. Furthermore, regulating market structure may mean restricting competition (where it is too costly e.g. involving too much duplicative capital spending; or where it is incapable of ensuring appropriate location of providers.

As I show in Part 3, there is a dissonance between New Labour's rhetoric of 'excess capacity to allow competition' and the reality of stringent cost-cutting in NHS hospitals. The question must be asked: would not direct public planning, with strategic management of resources, be more efficient as well as more equitable? In the US, piecemeal regulation discredited public planning in the 1970s, contributing to a conservative backlash (Paton, 1990). New Labour is not only amnesiac or ignorant of even the most recent decade in the UK, but susceptible only to good news from 'market systems'. In its economic naivety, it is in fact very Old Labour indeed (1920s-style).

The orthodoxy of the age is the government involved in 'steering but not rowing.' It is however an empirical question as to what works best. 'Positive regulation' usually involves a material incentive for the individual or organisation. 'Negative regulation' usually involves a sanction, whether material or otherwise. 'Arbitrative regulation' concerns a quasi-judicial process whereby criteria are set for the location, price, or quality of a service – with inspection and judgement carried out either by the regulator or a separate agency.

An obsession with 'steering and not rowing' can produce (unless government gives up on national standards, including equitable access) a labyrinthine 'post-modern' state...which does not demonstrate the inevitability of post-modernism or post-Fordist administrative structures so much as the pitfalls of designing policy in line with fashion.

A central tenet of new Labour's policy in 1997 was to 're-nationalise' the NHS so that services and access did not vary according to locality. The National Institute for Clinical Excellence was one manifestation of this. The government's policy also involved the prioritisation of services – e.g. cancer, cardiac care – which meant that delegation of generic 'needs – based' budgets to health authorities for local use was undermined in practice by national directives. In this context, why pretend that one is 'steering but not rowing'? It only leads to the mushrooming of agencies which have ephemeral powers.

The most pervasive example of the need for 'regulation' in the New Labour NHS is where it is absent – in the governance of local health 'economies'. Separate health agencies require effective criteria for either collaboration or competition – or for the domains of both – but instead 'duck and weave' from one temporary priority to another. 'Partnership' is preached to be a necessity, given the inter-dependence of agencies in meeting targets. Yet at non-executive level, securing agreement across local health economies on issues which are contentious is rendered difficult by policies which undermine cooperation. The reality is that the NHS is centrally-controlled; 'all the rest is embellishment and detail'. The 'hollowing out' of the state is a myth, yet the perpetuation of this myth has removed effective mechanisms for planning (e.g. regional service planning). Various strands of reform have promised 'devolution' and 'markets'. But the reality is more central control by the state than ever before because effective local planning has been disabled. Part 3 explores how this came about.

PART 3
The NHS

Chapter 6

Re-making the NHS

Those who cannot remember the past are condemned to repeat it

George Santayana

New Labour and Health Policy

If we date New Labour to the accession of Blair in 1994, we can see that the first frissons around health policy came from the fact that Blair's first Shadow Secretary of State for Health was Margaret Beckett. From the left of the party, she had entered parliament by defeating the right-wing Labour rebel Dick Taverne in 1974. She had become a junior Minister in the Callaghan government, but had then lost her seat at the 1979 election which brought Thatcher to power. In opposition she identified with the Bennite left, symbolised most notably by a coruscating attack on Neil Kinnock for abstaining, instead of supporting Tony Benn when the latter challenged the Deputy Leader Denis Healey in 1981.

She returned to parliament for a Derby seat in 1983, and has since then combined loyalty to the leadership with progressive principles. As Shadow Health Secretary, she mastered her brief well and was more convincing than her predecessor (who had moved on to Education), David Blunkett, who had kept policy analysis to a minimum, perhaps swallowing the clichés of the anti-doctor Left which were often not dissimilar to those of the anti-doctor Right. She was more in the tradition of Robin Cook, who (as Shadow Health Secretary from 1987 to 1992) had combined mastery of his brief with a lofty disdain for the Tories' confused policy – and had 'seen off' four Secretaries of State (Fowler, Moore, Clarke and Waldegrave).

But Blair's self-appointed task was to tack Right in health as elsewhere (some years later to embrace the 'new market', privatisation of elective surgery and increased role for the PFI – the latter to such an extent that he was attacked as too pro-PFI by Norman Lamont, the Tories' former Chancellor from the Eurosceptic Right of his party and architect of the PFI!). The issue of the PFI arose in those early days when Sheila Masters, who had been both on Conservative Prime Minister John Major's Private Finance panel and also senior partner with KPMG consultants, made a typically robust comment in 1995 claiming that Labour would change little in health policy, including PFI. With hindsight, one can see that it was possible that the Blairites had already put out feelers to the Right, given that there was later networking with think tanks that even the Conservatives had found too distant from the mainstream Right-of-centre.

Alerted to Masters'comments, Beckett 'slapped down' her presumptions and attacked the PFI. Within weeks she had been replaced as Shadow Secretary of State, and thereafter became a 'dignified' rather than 'official' part of the Labour leadership, to invoke the spirit of Bagehot.

Her successors in opposition were, respectively, Harriet Harman and Chris Smith, neither of whom made much impact. Both avoided controversy, which was a forerunner of the 1997 campaign approach that Labour's health policy was that it would 'save the NHS' ('100 days to save the NHS' was a prominent-election slogan).

It was convenient for New Labour, when approaching the health policy crossroads to 'signal left and turn right'. Whereas the Blairite strategy was to 'signal right' on the economy to avoid being tarred with the Old Labour brush, on the NHS people were more 'socialist' without thinking of it in those terms. Labour sounded 'anti-market' (in health, not in other areas) while clearly planning to retain the totem of the Tories' market, the 'purchaser/provider split'.

Perhaps one should say 'provide signals to both left and right'…the purchaser/ provider split was to be reinterpreted for the left (historically 'anti-doctor and anti-hospital' and 'pro-community healthcare') as a means to control hospitals and arrogant consultants; and maintained for the right as a symbol of New Labour's new managerialism if not yet its pro-market credentials (which had to wait until 2001)

Health policy pundits such as Chris Ham had provided legitimacy for the Tories' 1990s' NHS reforms. Ham had written a defence of the 'purchaser/provider split' in 1991 in the now-defunct 'Marxism Today'. Later, in 1995/6, when enthusiasm for the Tories' internal market was waning both in theory and practice, he sought to recast the pro-market 'narrative' as a 'pro primary care narrative'. Others stressed the taming of a traditional NHS elite and bogeyman (the 'barons' i.e. hospital consultants) rather than an ideological belief in competitive markets. Later Ham 'spun' the purchaser/ provider split (renamed the commissioner/provider separation) as a means for New Labour both to inherit the Thatcher reforms and to mould them (e.g. to abolish GP fund-holding yet maintain its ethos as regards 'taming hospitals').

'Commissioning' is ideally about defining needs and developing a strategy (including working with providers and developing them) in order to meet them, whereas purchasing is the more limited market transaction. Yet it was never thought through by New Labour (if it had been, it would have been seen to necessitate strategic planning – a very Soviet-sounding phrase for New Labour, in its paranoia about avoiding anything that sounded socialist.) Indeed one unintentionally humerous response, in an interview, by an NHS executive of the time went as follows: "apparently purchasing's out and commissioning's in… but we don't yet know what it is."

The usefulness of the 'pro primary care' spin (and more than spin) was that New Labour could genuflect to a long tradition on the left, embracing even a vulgar version of Marxism ('high technology medicine is just a sop to the workers given the absence of real public health') while maintaining the institutions (purchaser/provider splits and the like) which would later be useful in its own market reforms. This was both cock-up – or rather muddled thinking – and conspiracy.

The moderate left (such as Labour's first Secretary of State for Health after 1997, Frank Dobson) re-cast the purchaser into the form of the 'primary care group' (later trust i.e. PCT) but did not want to see market relations between purchaser and provider. To them the 'third way' (if such language must be used in an NHS context) meant collaboration in the cosy, local health family...or rather health economy, since families were thought to sound either twee or dysfunctional!

To the Blairites however, it was the left-sounding stuff that was spin – they wanted sincerely to preserve the NHS qua public funding, but they also had a Thatcherite belief both in 'bashing professions' (except lawyers, as with the lady herself) and in promoting market incentives – advised in particular by Simon Stevens (who made the ideological journey as adviser from Dobson to Blair via Milburn). Blair was later advised briefly by Julian le Grand, between October 2003 and early 2005 – the left-of-centre yet pro-market Richard Titmuss Professor of Health Policy (named in commemoration of the holder of the first Chair in Social Administration at the LSE. (Le Grand's prescriptions might well have had the eponymous Professor turning in his grave, although a chronological and ideological link of sorts was provided by Professor Brian Abel-Smith, Le Grand's predecessor, who became less hostile to the 1990s reforms shortly before his death in 1996.) Abel-Smith had advised Barbara Castle when she was Social Services Secretary (with responsibility for health) from 1974 to 1976.

In essence, the Blair government as it developed was interested in a 'reform' agenda which nevertheless had some 'dog whistles' for the Old Labour MPs on its back-benches. That meant, initially, treading carefully (just as Mrs. Thatcher had done in 1979 with the 'wets', whom she eventually outwitted and marginalized). Blair did the same with those of his cabinet who were not part of 'the project' (such as Frank Dobson at Health). But first there was an 'anti market' detour along the route of NHS reform.

Labour came into office saying that 'what counts is what works'. So what was the evidence for the various early approaches to re-organising the NHS?

Policy and Evidence

The Labour government's initial promise for the NHS was to 'cut the bureaucracy associated with the internal market.' Along with the modest target of reducing waiting-lists (not times) by 100,000, the party's manifesto had promised to cut management costs by £100million. This sort of promise is always vague. For a start, what are management costs? The Tories had claimed in the 1990s that the rise in management costs blamed on the market were partly due to reclassifying doctors and nurses and other clinicians as managers, and partly legitimate (i.e. the price of better management), although the latter claim was generally at management conferences as it was hardly a vote-winner! Now Labour might 'cut management costs' simply be 're-reclassifying' clinician-managers as clinicians!

Frank Dobson, the new Health Secretary, reacted angrily on the BBC Radio 4 Today programme in summer 1997 when informed that Nick Mays, a King's Fund analyst, had claimed that the NHS actually needed more, not less, investment in management. But this dispute was based on a confusion. There is a difference between the 'transactions costs' of the market, which are often administrative rather than managerial – or at least, tactical rather than strategic – and legitimate investment in management. It was the former which Dobson wanted to cut.

Additionally, while it may be true (even in 2006) that the NHS is 'over-administered and under-managed', the managerial investment now suggested to be in 1997 beneficial was in smaller 'primary care purchasing' (or commissioning) organisation. Research had suggested that, the more you spent on specialist purchasing (as in the 'Total Purchasing Pilot' organisations which had brought Fundholding GPs together with other local purchasers, in the dying years of the Tory government), the more effective it was – hardly an earth-shattering conclusion, and irrelevant to the wider question as to whether local purchasing **per se** was the right way to go.

More plausible is the view that it is large hospitals which require more, and better, middle and senior management – yet as part of an integrated health economy which eschews the 'divide and rule' of purchaser/provider splits.

It was with the latter that Dobson's heart lay, but no Blair government was about to abolish the purchaser/provider split. Ironically, Dobson nailed his colours to the shaky mast of the new Primary Care Groups (in essence an evolution from the 'Total Purchasing Pilots' rather than an innovation) as coordinators of care for communities. The rest is history: they became Primary Care Trusts (PCTs); they deepened conflict rather than the cooperation which Dobson had wanted, especially when 'Shifting the Balance of Power' (2001, see Part 2 above) came along, closely followed by the 'new market' after 2002.

It has been estimated that the PCT debacle – haltingly reversed in 2006 – cost well in excess of £1 billion in recurrent unnecessary management costs (Paton, 2006b). Add to this the direct costs of the new market ('Choose and Book'; Payment by Results' et al); the regulatory costs of the continuing targets regime; the costs of the 'new regulation' (see Chapter 5) and the costs to management of seeking local collaboration in such a hostile climate: in total, the costs of conflicting policies is arguably more than three times the national deficit of 2005-6. Ongoing 'reform' will indeed have to liberate huge efficiencies to recoup this, which could have been spent on patient care. As with the Conservative internal market, 'greater efficiency' is required to cover political embarrassment (ie cuts in hospitals to pay for the management overheads of policy).

And yet the 'evidence' which set in train the politics which led to the 'Shifting the Balance of Power' policy and to PCTs, covering small populations of about 100,000, came both from British evaluation of primary-care purchasing and from World Health Organisation prescription for natural communities of 100,000 – in a context far removed from England, and with no implication that such 'top heavy' managerial entities such as emerged in England could be or should be afforded. 'Evidence-based policy' is like Bernard Shaw's statistics (worse than damned lies) unless integrated with wider considerations and more strategic evidence. Yet most 'empirical evidence' in health policy and management is small-scale and technical. When one adds its capacity for being misunderstood – if (mis)used at all – by politicians rummaging for 'initiatives' in the garbage can, it should carry a health warning of the starkest sort.

Much health policy research 'evaluates' policy initiatives in technically sophisticated yet politically naïve ways. As just implied, a whole industry of research on 'primary care commissioning' between the 1990s and now has laboured to produce conclusions such as 'commissioners with a specialist interest in X generally commission services more effectively in the field of X' and 'the costs of (investing in and maintaining) commissioning are higher when commissioning is more ambitious...' Unfortunately this says nothing about the wider issue of whether these 'costs and benefits' are themselves commensurable with other consequences of 'local or primary' commissioning, and if so, how to adjudicate.

In a different way but at similar levels of naivety, the early empirical research on the 'internal market' (Robinson and le Grand (Eds.), 1994) implied that the first (voluntary) NHS 'Self-Governing' Trusts exhibited marginally higher productivity (by those limited official measures which were in place) than hospitals managed directly by the health authorities of the time. But this said nothing, or nothing new or analytical, even if true, about cause or effect (was it the 'better hospitals' according to official data which became Trusts – well of course it was! It was these hospitals which were politically chosen as the 'first-wave' Trusts).

Later research on the 1990s NHS 'market' (Le Grand, Mays and Mulligan, 1999) could take a wider sample over more years, and argued – in a useful, balanced report – that the evidence on the reforms as a whole was fairly equivocal. Regarding the above 'productivity' issue however, it was argued that the productivity growth in the NHS as a whole was a little higher in the 1990s than in preceding decades. If true, how could one distinguish between 'market incentives' and political 'command and control' as the reason – or indeed a host of other unquantifiable factors. The evidence, in other words, such as it was, was primitive.

Similarly, recent study of the four UK health systems post-1997 (and post–1999 devolution) implies that England – has achieved higher activity rates than Scotland, Wales and Northern Ireland, in terms of cutting waiting times (Alvarez-Rosete et al, 2005). Here, there is a major additional problem to add to that outlined above: what is the time lag between a policy regime and improved service? Up until 2003, the market was not operative (PCTs only came into existence nationally in England by 2002, and their 'purchasing' was 'steady-state' in 2002-3.) So it is in fact the 'central command and control' of the Milburn years, which chivvied the English NHS to pull up its socks, which is actually responsible for the improvements.

This is not a Luddite suggestion that we ignore evidence: it is a reminder of its lethal nature if it is taken out of context or assembled with an implicit model of 'politics' as external rather than integral.

The Levels of Policy

The three Parts of this book are intended to depict policy at different levels. Part 1 shows the external environment of political economy and its major influence (and constraint) upon policy. Part 2 builds political economy into a hierarchy of factors which must be viewed 'separately yet together' in explaining policy – and especially how apparently countervailing pressures on policy (political economy, at one extreme; day-to-day 'initiatives and agendas', on the other hand) have to be reconciled.

The present Part 3 presents the 'view from the bunker' (or at least from the engine-room) rather than the view from the bridge. How does policy, as explained in Parts 1 and 2, actually appear, and feel, 'on the ground'; and how consistent or otherwise is it in meeting the strategic service objectives which it must meet?

New Labour's dilemma is its perception that it is 'swimming against the tide' in seeking to save the NHS, and its resulting but ironical obsession with persistent re-organisation. This increasingly emphasises 'GP commissioning' and also the new market of 'patient choice.' These are not the same thing; indeed they are alternatives. Real patient choice would remove the relevance of commissioning (in the sense of contracts with providers by commissioners). Currently New Labour is vitiating the incentives of 'patient choice buttressed by payment of results' – its 'showroom' policy – by restricting the flows of money into hospitals (which is what patients tend to choose!) though its 'backdoor' policy of limiting hospital income in line with restrictive contracts.

New Labour has made a rod for its own back. It expects 'instant results' (for example, panics when new money has failed to improve productivity within two years, despite this being unrealistic.) It is a victim of its own 'post-modern' approach to the media and spin. Sir Humphrey Appleby would have advised New Labour to be more cautious with its targets, so that they could be met! Admittedly the government has sought to 'stretch' the NHS in order to increase patient satisfaction, which is admirable, while some targets, are of the Sir Humphrey variety. But it is less the formal targets (although these are now much more ambitious than the fatuous pledge-card variety of 1997) than the general expectations as to productivity which is the problem. On the latter, the government has accepted the diagnosis, and criteria, of both the market think tanks and 'official bodies' (such as the Office of National Statistics and the OECD) which are often too aggregated to be meaningful.

Below are provided some selective illustrations of how 'ideas' (usually based on ideology) work out in practice. This includes an examination of the 'new market' in healthcare, on the grounds that it is New Labour's 'big idea' from its second and third terms in government, and the criterion (as a major part of 'public sector reform') on which Blair wishes his legacy to be judged. This includes consideration of how the 'theory' of choice (mostly from economics) is affected by politics, with reference to the arguments of the Albert Hirschman (1970) in his classic work.

Ideas often matter, 'on the ground'. But this is less for the 'positive' – the academic elegance of their assumptions, and the attractiveness to politicians of the blueprints they offer – than for the 'negative', the ways in which they can have unforeseen or counter-productive consequences when applied in particular contexts.

Ideas find publicity, even if not meaningful implementation, when they accord with the dominant ideology. In the 1980s, the NHS reform agenda was about 'managerialism' but not (yet) markets. In this context, rationing (by 'experts') was a major theme which was in tune with the spirit of the age. The 1960s and 1970s had gone; expansion and consensus were 'yesterday's approach.' Resources had to be applied better. 'QALYs' researchers, who had developed 'Quality Adjusted Life Years as the yardstick for judging treatments in healthcare, provided the spirit of the age.

Then came the era of the 'market Phase 1' in which micro-economists held sway, with their models of (public sector) markets. Then we had the transition time of the 1990s, when the Conservative government was eventually seen to be on the way out, and the Blair government was waiting in the wings. What would actually happen in healthcare was unclear, both in terms of levels of expenditure and the nature of the system (would it be 'trust the professionals' or continue with the Tories' reforms?) This was the age of the pragmatic pundit. And subsequently we have the 'era of the 'market Phase 2' but with a wider political and academic base than the 'economist's market' of the early 1990s. 'We are all marketers now', it seems.

In other words, it is important to cast a critical eye over 'ideas', to explore how they interact with politics and political management.

Idea 1 – 'Primary Care Good, Hospital Bad'

There is a strong strain of thinking which is convenient to New Labour, in that it fulfils the agenda of sounding 'progressive', Old Labour and even socialist, while also promoting the New Labour agenda of markets and managerialism. That is the 'pro primary care, anti-hospital' strain allowing a convergence of the 'vulgar Marxist' view of 'high-technology medicine as elitist' (Navarro, 1978) with the pro-market agenda of squeezing hospitals. What's more, Labour can say things like, 'if the miners were disciplined by the market, why shouldn't the 'elite' such as the hospital barons also be disciplined?' – which goes down well with their 'poor bloody infantry' required on the door-knocker at election time.

As a result of this strain, which strongly influenced Labour Health Secretary Patricia Hewitt through her association with the Institute for Public Policy Research (IPPR) and no doubt provided a cognitive link for this loyal Blairite to her radical leftist past, just as it had associated Conservative Health Secretary Virginia Bottomley with a community orientation in the 1990s, hospitals are depicted as 'milking' the budget. They therefore require to be cut down to size (as with the 2006 policy; see Stage 5 of the 'garbage can, Part 2 above.) Yet the reality is if anything the opposite. Hospitals are being squeezed by dogma rather than by evidence.

Inconsistency

Admittedly the policy of Payment by Results, introduction from 2005-6 – if allowed to operate in pure form – would ensure that hospitals were 'paid what they deserved', for treating patients which PCTs (actually, GPs) could not keep out of hospital through effective primary care. In fact the policy of PBR was designed and 'sold' to Ministers on one of their other (competing) agendas – that of providing a rigorous approach to market forces which did not allow competition on the basis of price, as in the Tory 1990s market. Price competition has its defenders (Donaldson and Ruta, 2005) but it was brought into disrepute in the 1990s (Propper et al, 2004). Nevertheless PBR did not help the 'anti-hospital, pro-primary care, pro-'community services' agenda – it was plucked out of the garbage can for a different purpose by a different Health Secretary, and inherited by Hewitt (who privately wondered about reining it in).

So the policy has been 'toughened', by arbitrarily cutting the tariff (prices set nationally for different treatments) for admissions to hospital, especially emergencies – even when 'primary care' cannot keep the patients away from either A and E or actual admission. This of course encourages price competition by the backdoor, as hospitals able and willing to do this work for less will be more viable in the market. And so the dangers of a market based on price competition, in terms of clinical quality and even mortality rates arise again, with New Labour's 'learning' from the Conservative market apparently unlearnt.

Along with this went the 'scapegoating' of hospitals at a time when, embarrassingly for New Labour, the whole NHS was in deficit by at least £1billion despite the undoubted extra resources it had received – and largely because of policy enactments by government, including the mushrooming of uncoordinated primary care organisations. It is convenient to imply that all deficits are the result of bad management or leadership, or high costs due to services not having been 'reconfigured.' The reality is very different. (Paton, 2006 d)

Deficits: Using a Crisis to Downsize Hopitals?

The size of financial deficits in the NHS, despite significant new investment and expenditure since 2001, received widespread attention in the media from the end of 2005 onwards (Guardian, 2005). A wide range of factors was responsible for deficits in various NHS Trusts, Primary Care Trusts and also Foundation Trusts. Some of these factors were related to the government's 'new market' reforms but most were not – as the main reforms only began in 2006. Some factors were 'supply side' (such as workforce reforms and higher pay); and some were 'demand (including national targets; stimulation of the private sector by central government; and the whole raft of government initiatives since the NHS plan, especially the expensive Shifting the Balance of Power but also including the other key – and conflicting – policy strands.) The government's reform agenda since 1997 has contained many policy strands prior to the 'new market' per se, such as new structures and roles for commissioning; new standards (and targets); and revived approaches to cooperation within 'local health economies', despite the market. It was convenient for government to ascribe all deficits to inefficiency or poor management, given the post-Wanless (2002) levels of investment in the NHS. It is important however to separate out the different causes of deficits around the country, which are widespread but not homogeneous, to distinguish between the intended and unintended effects of policy, structural factors across the NHS and factors internal to Trusts (including the early consequences of 'payment by results' as well as endemic inefficiency.) Poor implementation of an over-loaded policy agenda may well lead to 'the wrong providers closing' (or contracting) ie the wrong culprit being 'reconfigured', and the political destabilisation of the English NHS. The emergence of a national deficit by April 2006, which was around five times that which the Secretary of State had believed it to be only three months before, coincided with the government's initiative to make a radical shift of care in the community. As a result, hospital Trusts with large deficits were 'targeted' for radical contraction (sometimes called 'efficiency') whatever the cause of deficits – whether or not community services were ready , able or willing to take up the slack (Paton, 2006e). This was all the more ironical if and when the inability of PCTs to pay for patients they could not treat in primary settings was the cause of deficit.

The Supply Side

On the 'supply side', five factors loom large. They are: the cost of implementing Agenda for Change, the government's workforce reform programme; the cost of the new Consultant contract; the cost of the new GP contract; the continuing costs of compliance with the European Working Time Directive; and the locally-borne share of the government's ambitious IM and T programme.

More than half of the 'new money' for the NHS has gone on pay. About half of this is for new staff; about half is related to the above labour force reforms. This is often presented pejoratively, but recruitment and retention in a global economy must be taken seriously. It was always the case that the costs of reform would 'kick' in before benefits, and the current 'moral panic' about costs is partly exacerbated by the absence of a realistic timetable for predicted benefits and the predictable 'panic' by government when the media hits hard. The government is good at plucking reforms out of the 'garbage can' of ideas but poor at implementation.

Much recent criticism stems from an alleged falling or stagnant productivity in the English NHS. But it may be asked: if staff numbers and pay are increased quickly, what else can one expect? Again, even Trusts in the middle of 'efficiency drives' and (for example) 'three year financial recovery plans' were suddenly targeted for urgent action with wheels being reinvented wholesale, as prescriptions for eg radical reductions in length of stay were soon seen to require massive investment in primary and community care – the absence of which was often responsible for hospital deficits in the first place, as hospitals were forced to treat many more cases than the PCTs had 'modelled' in their budgets. Some defenders of the ideas of the 'new market' in the English NHS point out that the latter is allegedly performing better than the Welsh and Scottish NHSs. They seem to want have it both ways: incipient benefits in England can be ascribed to market forces but problems are to be ascribed to the absence of market forces. In any case, the 'new market' only began in 2006: the improvement in England (Alvarez-Rosete et al, *op. cit*) was due to central performance management at the height of central command!

The Demand Side

On the 'demand' side, many factors loomed large in explaining financial pressure. Positively, many NHS Trusts had sought – in response to government urging – to tackle both overt and hidden waiting times (the latter including MRI and CT scans as well as cardiology procedures), so that overall average waits as well as headline targets were addressed. This was generally encouraged pre-election in 2005, whereas after 2006, 'minimal targets and no more' were the order of the day at the Department of Health – except in the Prime Minister's rhetoric about meeting the 2008 targets (Paton, 2006b). For hospital staff, this is often demotivating as well as confusing – but it is patients, with some categories of operations now cancelled en bloc, who matter most. The achievement of the Prime Ministers personal target of "18 weeks from GP consultation to hospital discharge" was thereby put in serious doubt.

Explanations for financial pressures on the demand side also include the role of the private sector: centrally-mandated monies for Independent Sector Treatment Centres (allocated broad brush) reduce allocations to PCT's at the local level; and 'out-sourcing' of operations more generally is necessary locally due to lack of NHS capacity in some areas of the country. One should add, when considering the private sector, a factor which may be considered both 'supply' and 'demand': those providers with large Private Finance Initiatives have to bear both large transitional 'accounting costs' (such as impairment of existing capital) and also an interest rate (to reimburse the borrowing costs and also profits of the private partner) which may be almost double the public sector 'capital charge' (which has been reduced from 6% to 3.5%) which determines the funding flow to providers for capital charges. This is actually a supply-side (capital) cost, but is accounted by the Treasury as a revenue issue, for reasons to do with keeping the Chancellor's macro-economic promises about borrowing (the 'golden rule') rather than health policy.

The rising tide of emergency admissions and A and E consultations reflects the fact that a 'primary care led' NHS is rhetoric but not reality. GPs work less 'out of hours' than ever, for example, as a result of their new contract overtly recognising their unwillingness so to do. This is despite large extra income to meet 'quality' standards which arguably should be intrinsic. Where PCTs have not coordinated effective local action to keep the chronically ill from regular presentation at the acute hospital, hospitals may find that they are swamped by emergencies. From 2006, the latter are only partially reimbursed 'at tariff' through the Payment by Results policy (PBR) in an attempt to limit costs. In other words, 'demand management' is being sought through desperate actions, implemented piecemeal. Emergencies will still be paid by 'block contract' (if local haggling over contracts can be dignified by that name), which may seriously underestimate reasonable costs. Meanwhile there may ironically be less space in the hospital for those elective admissions which are paid at tariff…which may indeed not happen in practice, if the PCTs cannot afford to do so and therefore restrict the volume they will pay for through 'contracts' which undermine any real notion of patient choice. To describe it as 'managed choice' is a euphemism. The difference between a budget deficit and 'bad debt' is a nicety in which NHS regulators tend not to be interested.

Commissioning and Structural Factors

The configuration of commissioning since Shifting the Balance of Power was rightly recognised to be dysfunctional by the government – hence its July 2005 document, Commissioning A Patient-Led NHS. In the meantime, political compromises in the latter's implementation by a weakened government, fighting a rearguard action in education as well as health, allowed backbenchers to defend existing local PCT fiefdoms – described in Part 2 above as a kind of pork-barrel politics without the pork (local MPs are often unknowingly arguing for the local right to delay operations or deny care, in arguing for the retention of their local health agencies autonomy). In many parts of England, commissioning is rather like Western civilisation, according to Mahatma Gandhi – a nice idea, which will never happen! For hospitals, this can spell the difference between solvency and deficit – more the outcome of the visible fist than the invisible hand. (See the analysis of choice and the new market below)

Commissioning a Patient-Led NHS suggested Practice-Based Commissioning (PBC) – to give GPs an incentive to 'repatriate' out-patient follow up, and to seek to get the alleged benefits of the 1990s policy of GP Fundholding without the costs. Donaldson and Ruta (*op. cit*) argue for a model of 'superpractices', with patients choosing which of these to which to belong, rather than which hospital to attend. The reality however, as with the more tightly-financed US managed care, is that the patient would end up following the contract rather than exercising choice. PBC or 'managed care English-style' cuts across the GP's role as honest broker for the patient in exercising choice. It merely devolves the conflict of interest which the PCT was rightly identified as having (between commissioning and provision) to practice or 'superpractice' level.

It would be better to fund integrated local health economies, with allocations adjusted in line with patient choice of elective procedures. This would allow strategic planning of specialised and emergency or urgent services, performance management and yet choice for patients where appropriate – with the 'hospital/community' dividing line established by clinical need and not dogma. It is more than twenty years ago that Sir Douglas Black described the 'acute/primary' divide as a "false antithesis". (Black, 1984).

Even more reprehensibly, it is politically and managerially convenient to 'concentrate' deficits within the large acute hospital Trust. Then they can be passed off as 'bad apples in a healthy barrel'. This is convenient to Ministers: the challenge is perceived – wrongly – as a managerial problem of 'sorting out bad apples' rather than a political and structural problem. The managerial 'fixers' are at regional (Strategic Health Authority) level, and they earn their rewards by imposing simplistic solutions on (mostly) hospitals.

Yet deficits are generally spread over the whole 'health economy', not just hospitals; as just described, hospital deficits often result from 'bad debt' in that PCTs do not pay properly for their patients admitted to hospital, in order to husband their own resources for their own 'sectional' priorities (see Part 2, Political Institutions under New Labour) and of course to avoid or minimise their own deficits. About three quarters of the agencies in deficit at the end of 2005-6 were hospitals – the real picture would attribute many of these deficits to PCTs. The 'spin' was that '50% of deficits were in 7% of institutions' (and rising!). But what about the other 50%? And, if deficits were correctly ascribed to source it would be more like, 50% in 25% of institutions; a meaningless statistic, or rather one which emphasises the salience of the problem.

The idea of 'hospital bad, primary/community good' can do a lot of damage when combined with political and economic realities. Crucially, good hospitals can be undermined or even destroyed by tactics encouraged by the practical import of the prevailing ideology 'primary care needs more money; hospitals less'. The purchaser/ provider split was overtly justified as a means of changing priorities (away from the hospital) as well as improving efficiency. It has not done the latter (Paton et al, 1998).

And as regards the former, New Labour is discovering that 'local commissioning' undermines the national nature and vision of the NHS – what you get depends on your postcode, especially at times of financial stress. Herceptin, and the tragic stories across the country about differential access to a drug whose assessment NICE was 'fast tracking' in 2006, is a clear example of confusion – and of Ministers trying to have it both ways. On the one hand, it is 'local decision' (without extra resources); on the other hand Ministers make urgent telephone calls to 'direct' that it should be prescribed...to some PCT Chairs but not others, depending on the politics of (literally) the day. Herceptin, for early-stage breast cancer, may or may not be suitable for pre-authorisation prescription in all cases; what is more, the story is a complicated one and demonstrates both irrationality in policy and decision-making, on the one hand, and 'pressure group' politics (albeit of the must understandable kind) in allocating NHS resources.

The real point here, however, is that the cocktail of both 'local commissioning' and 'anti-hospital spin' is damaging both to coherent policy and to the prospects for a humane and understandable approach to priority-setting in the NHS.

Summary

The idea of a 'primary care bias' is as old as the twentieth century. It was especially convenient to New Labour, as it wished to preserve the NHS institutions it inherited from the Conservatives in 1997, while advertising their use for 'holistic primary care'. Although the NHS Plan of 2000 (briefly) recommended *de facto* investment in hospitals and the choice/PBR policy created an (unintentional) 'hospital bias', policy has now been rationalised to 'go for broke' in the community. There has indeed been a trend in this direction, running from New Labour's first White Paper on the NHS (Department of Health, 1997), through StBoP (2001), to 'Our Health, Our Care, Our Say (DoH, 2006).

And yet it is typical that confusion (and deficits) caused by policy incompatibilities was the 'opportunity' to re-establish the 'anti-hospital' strategy. That is: the strategy had been lost in the maelstrom of 'events' and its re-emergence was not as a result of evidence or need but as a means of rationalising a crisis.

Idea 2 – Decentralisation

Shifting the Balance of Power' (StBoP, 2001) was based on the idea of 'decentralisation' – in fact it was called 'devolution', but the latter implies political power at a lower level, which did not occur. I have explored the 'problem with PCTs' in Part 2 above, as part of the story of how politics and health organisations are mutually embedded at the local level. The other key element of StBoP was the creation of Strategic Health Authorities (SHAs) to replace Regions – which were actually useful and appropriately-sized, but 'sounded' bureaucratic, so had to go. The SHAs as created in 2001/2 were dysfunctional and only lasted three to four years – longer than the 'Regional Directorates of Health and Social Care (DHSCs), created at the same time to oversee the SHAs, which were abolished before they had found premises!

Strategic Health Authorities have often failed to act strategically in reconfiguring hospital services in their areas, as well as PCTs. This is in part out of subservience to Ministers' fears of 'local politics', despite their brave words about 'markets' and 'tough management'; in part, because their remit is weak and indirect (a major flaw of their creation); and in part, because many SHA executives and Chairs are apparatchiks rather than independent public servants. As good apparatchiks, their talent is often in the psychology of the 'kiss up, kick down' culture.

SHAs, in accordance with the variant of institutional rational choice theory known as 'bureau shaping' theory (Dunleavy, 1991), have an interest in maximising their power and influence while minimising their 'hands on' responsibility. Thus they tend to monitor performance rather than manage it. For example, they leave it to NHS Trusts and PCTs to seek local agreements – yet devolve blame to them if they fail to do so – rather than take the lead in developing strategy for their areas and thereby helping to reconfigure both providers and commissioners (thereby linking service strategy with financial strategy). Indeed, as ever, national initiative was required (Commissioning a Patient-Led NHS, 2005) to sort out local messes, where there were too many small and often incompetent PCTs, and the wrong configuration of hospital services.

SHAs, unlike the Regional Offices they replaced in 2001, are officially NHS bodies rather than outposts of the Department of Health (DoH.) Yet in reality they are in a 'no man's land' between the two: they are supposed to be 'facilitative' and 'developmental' for the NHS, yet the way in which the Department of Health 'performances manages' them (as NHS bodies themselves) encourages classic 'apparatchik' behaviour.

'Deficits Again': Using Crisis to Enforce Central Control Under the Guise of 'Regulation'

A classic example of 'apparatchik' behaviour – as opposed to independent-mindedness and creative planning – was found in SHAs' reaction to the Secretary of State for Health's 'panic' about NHS deficits in Financial Year 2005-6. Firstly, there was an attempt to paint them as isolated examples. SHAs, keen to 'kiss up' to the DoH, at first under-reported deficits (partly out of ignorance of the reality in their 'patches'; partly on desperately optimistic assumptions, or rather optimistically desperate assumptions!) such that the DoH reported the national total for England in December to be £200million. By February it was £600million. By the time Sir Nigel Crisp resigned as PS and CE of the NHS on March 7th, it had reached £750million. Ten days later it was £850 million and rising. By the end of April, it was estimated to be £1.2 billion.

By this stage, as remarked above, the story was that '50% of the deficit total was in 7% of the organisations'. SHAs sought to point to 'isolated'(if big) deficits – yet the reality was often underlying deficits spread over hospital NHS Trusts and PCTs (see above). These were often disguised by PCTs 'passing the buck' to NHS Trusts.

There is now a real problem in the NHS of 'bad policy resulting in the loss of good management', rather than just 'bad management resulting in deficits' But Ministers were in denial. Their answer to deficits was therefore 'Department of Health turnaround teams'. By now, the new market era was beginning, and many hospitals were being 'diagnosed' as potential Foundation Trusts, with Monitor (the NHS economic 'regulator'; see conclusion to Part 2 above) in charge of developing individual NHS Trusts for 'foundation status. This consisted in 'greater fitness for purpose' for survival in the new NHS market. So SHAs, Monitor (and 'turnaround teams') all had a role in examining Trusts – with conflict of interest between development purposes, on the one hand, and performance assessment, on the other hand, put on one side.

Instead of seeking a consistent approach between themselves geared to the coherence (in service terms) of whole 'health economies' (i.e. areas of about half a million, within SHAs and wider in the case of specialised services and clinical networks generally), piecemeal approaches were adopted. A key example of the latter was the search for radically-shortened lengths-of-stay in hospital, yet – in the very same health economy – PCTs being advised to cut their 'community beds'. This meant not only that the Health Secretary's latest initiative ('Our Health, Our Care, Our Say, 2006), which called for expanded community facilities, was undermined by her own turnaround teams, but that radically shortening lengths-of-stay was either impossible or potentially catastrophic for patients.

Labour had announced, on taking office in 1997, both a 'bed closure moratorium' (in that too many beds had been lost in the 1990s on 'heroic' planning assumptions, often made by management consultancies (Leys, 1999)) and a rule that new 'PFI hospitals' should not lead to a net bed reduction. The latter was however fudged in that 'beds outside hospital' could be counted yet often there was no mechanism to ensure that they were kept open by PCTs or available for general use of the wider health economy as opposed to the individual PCT – another problem with the ultra-fragmented NHS post-2001. By 2006, these safeguards were in freefall, and PFI schemes were being radically 'downsized' – with heroic assumptions about reduced use of hospitals being made.

That is, both of these policies were undermined in the 2005-6 financial panic (the former already had been), as was the rule that occupancy of hospitals should not be planned, in new developments, to be more than 84%. This was based on international good practice, and was useful for flexibility and quality as well as crucial for safety in the era of MRSA and other 'superbugs.'

The crucial point is that such reversal of good practice was driven nationally, by new guidelines and 'turnaround teams' rather than by decentralized responsibility in the new 'decentralized' NHS.

'Turnaround'

In terms of national /local balance: a typical 'deficit Trust' might play host to all or any:

(1) the national turnaround team;

(2) the Foundation Trust 'diagnostics' team (SHA-led, with Monitor representation, and often different agendas within the joint team);

(3) an SHA 'advisory panel';

(4) an SHA Board observer;

(5) a 'personal help to the Acting Chief Executive' hired from a consultancy firm;

(6) a national accountancy consultancy hired to advise on cost-recovery (likely to come up with striking recommendations such as 'greater cooperation with PCTs' as well as heroic assumptions about matters such as length-of-stay (see above);

(7) a health-economy-wide cost-recovery team – separate from (6) above;

(8) internal auditors;

(9) external auditors.

Clearly not all of these are the responsibility of the SHA, although most are. All are charge-able to the 'host' trust, with the exception of (4) above. The list does not 'prove' anything: it can be acknowledged that 'turnaround' focuses upon 'problem' organisations (or rather, those defined as such). But the symbolic effect on the rest of the NHS should not be lost: it is, 'here's the agaenda'; here's what Monitor expects; play the game this way or else.' It also suggests an approach which is both 'control freak' and yet scattergun – worryingly geared to the 'turnaround' of an individual organisation rather than to an appreciation of structural factors, including national policy. The SHA's role is to react to problems, in order to 'report up' to the Department of Health, which is notoriously coy at reporting other than good news to Ministers. Strikingly the NHS's financial regime for 'turnaround' is now crippling. The so-called 'double whammy' means that Trusts have to reduce expenditure by twice their deficit (however caused): firstly, to reduce the deficit; and secondly, to pay it back in one year. Despite the Secretary of State for Health announcing under pressure in March 2006 on the BBC's *Panorama* that this regime would be reviewed, the Secretary of State for Health and Prime Minister have since insisted that it is the basis for 'turning around' the NHS.

Most importantly, such an account shows that rhetoric suggesting a culture of decentralization in the NHS is a smokescreen. We have seen a persistent cycle from 'devolution to centralism' in the NHS (Paton, 1993). Yet the reality has been growing centralism since 1982, even in the era of the new market. Private sector involvement has been another reason for this: (again, in opposition to prevailing rhetoric) the political reality of 'enticing' the private sector into the NHS is centrally-devised incentives and directives, imposed on the local NHS.

We have seen this phenomenon with 'Independent Sector Treatment Centres' used for 'Fast-track' treatments under national initiatives. More significantly, the Private Finance Initiative (PFI) has necessitated tight central control by the Treasury (in general through its high-level PFI advisers and advocates; in particular through its Capital Investment Branch). The PFI has also led to greater centralism in project-approval in the Department of Health, and its Private Finance Unit.

Such project planning is actually the essence of health service planning, although concealed as 'technical monitoring'. Despite the rhetoric about local commissioning, 'he who controls the capital does the planning.' Capital is privately-supplied by PFI consortia (or rather, by the financial sector via PFI consortia to the public sector, with two expensive middlemen by comparison with publicly-financed capital). This is simply to keep public capital off the 'Public Sector Debt' register. The PFI is explored further below.

Recently New Labour Ministers have become concerned about the cost and inflexibility of 'PFI hospitals', in the context of the 2005-6 'deficit crisis', despite initially accepting the PFI hook, line and sinker after the removal of Margaret Beckett from her Shadow Health portfolio in 1995. The trouble is that PFI schemes must have either high cost or inflexibility. Leaving schemes 'flexible', with the private sector responsible for initial design and response to later public-sector changes in requirements, means huge cost. Stipulating in detail the public sector's requirements can reduce cost to some extent – but in effect means the NHS doing the design and detailed specification, with the private sector's only real role (other than contracting to build and run, which does not require PFI-type financing) being to raise the money more expensively than could the Treasury, if it so wished.

It is factors such as these which make 'decentralisation' a chimera. There is, despite the rhetoric of 'devolution from the centre, overseen by external regulation', a top-heavy interventionist culture in the NHS. Sadly, this does not realise the potential advantage of centralism (coherent planning) but the disadvantage (arbitrary or piecemeal interventions). When one adds to the mechanisms for external assurance of internal control and external assurance of external control (Scrivens, 2005) both direct political control and indirect political control posing as external regulation (as with Monitor – see Chapter Seven), the reality is an over-politicised NHS in which regulatory fragmentation allows politicians to 'divide and rule' among the so-called regulators.

At least, if political control is inevitable, it would be honest to admit this and cut the waste and bureaucracy involved in the panoply of agencies required to perpetuate the myth of the 'new governance'.

Summary

Much of the rhetoric around New Labour's health policy has involved devolution and/or decentralisation . The New NHS: Modern and Dependable (DoH, 1997) stressed the role of the (then) Primary Care Groups (PCGs), in organising integrated local care. StBoP, with the PCGs successor Primary Care Trusts (PCTs), continued to stress the 'front line' rather than 'managers' – although by now the 'commissioner/ provider split' was alive and well again in Minister's minds. Subsequent rhetoric, in Next Steps for Investment, Next Steps for Reform (DoH, 2002) and all the other harbingers of the 'new market', stressed choice and markets (without using the word) rather than devolution – and indeed they are different concepts.

The organisation of a market within public services tends to lead to central control (Paton et al, 1998), a lesson Labour forgot from less than ten years before. Additionally, the tension between New Labour's aspirations for a **national** service (as with NICE, and national service frameworks) and its 'localising' rhetoric meant that – as in the 1990s – 'localism' was in fact local responsibility for doing national bidding, rather than local power.

The next 'idea' examined is 'private involvement in the NHS' per se.

Idea 3 – Private Management

Private management is defined here in three senses: the privatisation of healthcare provision, with private management of private companies; the private management of public providers; and the peculiarly British policy of the PFI, introduced above, which is a vehicle for major capital schemes which the Treasury wishes to keep 'off balance sheet' but which also has long-term implications for introducing partially-private management into the running of 'NHS hospitals.'

Regarding the first – privatisation of provision – the argument 'for' is generally one of technical efficiency. New Labour has sought to 'shake up' both the public sector and the traditional, home-based private sector by injecting competition. This new impetus is paradoxically driven by central command from the Department of Health, rather than by local choice of NHS 'purchasers' or 'commissioners' of care, the Primary Care Trusts (PCTs) –although there is a small-scale tradition of 'contracting out': support services (dating from 1983); specific clinical services (eg 'at the margin', to help with the reduction of waiting lists and times in line with central government policy); and to traditional private, not-for-profit providers (eg of specialist mental health care).

The new drive is to recruit privately-managed companies, especially from abroad, employing either imported staff or (former or part-time) NHS staff. The so-called 'ISTCs' – Independent Sector Treatment Centres' – are the major plank of this policy. They deal with short-stay 'elective' healthcare (eg in ophthalmology (cataracts) and orthopaedics (hips). Another trend in England in particular is to contract with private companies in order to import 'management models' and actual private management for particular conditions – including particular chronic diseases and even general 'community services' such as post-hospital nursing and overall 'client care'. A prominent example is United Health Care, Europe (including its 'Evercare' model) whose European President is Simon Stevens, until recently Health Adviser to Tony Blair the British PM.

The main argument 'con' is four-fold (with the first two general and the latter two more specific to England today.) Firstly, there are worries that integrated care may be more difficult to organise if, instead of integrated public provision, a plurality of providers with different incentives and cultures have to be 'managed' in providing services to patients and clients. Secondly, the private sector may be a 'Trojan horse' – in that short-term 'efficiency gains' may be bought at the cost of relative disinvestment in NHS facilities. As a result, private providers may be able to 'call the shots' with public payers in the longer term. Thirdly, means of costing and reimbursing providers may disadvantage the residual NHS providers – who are left with the 'heavy duty' work of both emergency and specialised varieties yet whose reimbursement depends upon spreading 'fixed costs' over the 'whole hospital portfolio', some of which they have now lost. Fourthly, the official policy and rhetoric about creating enough capacity so that both private and public sectors can flourish in a 'new choice-driven market' is now being undermined by the need to solve NHS financial deficits by restricting public capacity (yet financing the private sector generally).

Regarding my second category – private management of public providers – the main argument 'pro' is the improvement of 'failing organisations' in the public sector without privatising them. The forms this policy has recently taken in the UK have been the formal 'franchising' of the management of (a small number of) NHS hospitals in England (again, with the process controlled by central government), on the one hand, and the informal insertion of 'private managers' to join public management teams in hospitals which remain publicly governed.

The former was much heralded from 2002, but has remained insignificant in practice. The English NHS has witnessed the latter on a large scale towards the end of 2005 – in response to systemic financial deficits across the acute hospital sector – in the form of 'turnaround teams', some of which will have a long-term presence in hospitals. These teams are mostly from the large and often multi-national accountancy/consultancy firms. Additionally, NHS authorities (such as the Strategic Health Authorities, situated between the Department of Health and localities) often place 'cronies' (usually former NHS managers now working as private consultants) at the right-hand of NHS Chief Executives.

The main argument 'con' is two-fold. Firstly, apart from the exorbitant cost, the concern is that such 'targeted' management prioritises financial savings in individual hospitals in a fragmented manner, without taking the bigger picture into account. The resulting configuration of clinical services across both localities and wider areas may involve both overlap and omission (especially of specialised services, which are often an 'easy target' – being both expensive and involving relatively small numbers). Secondly, 'external private managers and advisers' may have little regard to the culture of organisations, and so short term successes may be counterbalanced by long term problems.

Regarding my third category, the Private Finance Initiative (PFI) is a mechanism by which private consortia – usually formed specially to contract with private design, construction, equipment and management firms – develop and run new hospitals (including management of everything apart from direct clinical services) in return for a long-term 'revenue' income stream from the public sector (ie the 'unitary payment', over an agreed time-period of often thirty-five years, comprising: the 'payback' for the capital they had to borrow; profit; and the 'cost-plus' of equipping and managing the hospital for the agreed period.)

The PFI began as a 'public sector wide' policy in 1990 when Norman Lamont was Chancellor of the Exchequer in the Conservative government. Subsequently, after a hiatus (see beginning of this Chapter), New Labour widened and deepened the policy.

The main arguments are as follows. Firstly, it is a policy of 'jam today, pay tomorrow.' This may be seen as either a 'pro' or a 'con'. For politicians who want to 'bring home the bacon' now and postpone costs until they have left the scene, it is a 'pro'! In terms of cost-effectiveness, it may be a 'con'. Until recently English Health Ministers held the line that the policy was efficient, in that risk associated with new developments was transferred to the private sector. Recently however this has been suggested to be an illusion, as the Treasury is the payer of last resort. Additionally, the cost of transferring risk (ie getting the private sector to be willing to bear it, plus paying it the requisite profit – which has been arranged most uncompetitively at 'cost plus') has been exorbitant.

The main point of the policy has been to keep capital expenditure 'off the government's balance sheet' ie it has not been a policy deriving from the specific needs of the health sector but a generic macro-economic/accounting sleight-of-hand.

Until recently, an argument 'pro' the PFI would have been that more new hospitals could be financed this way than government of any political hue could have allowed using public money. But the government is now belatedly realising that the policy may be both a 'bad deal' financially and a source of inflexibility in the long term (with the Department of Health's Head of Capital Planning criticising the tendency to build 'monuments'). Ironically this had been Labour's stance in opposition pre-1995, to a policy developed by the previous Conservative government). As a result it has been 'paring back' PFI schemes before 'financial close' (ie formal contract between the NHS and the private consortium after both 'commercial close' and the acquisition of finance from the money markets).

Another argument 'pro' has been the alleged conservatism and slowness of the public sector in managing new hospital schemes. It is argued that the PFI 'boxes in public managers' by a formal contract for new facilities ie prevents them reneging on their own plans when finances or time gets tight! Unfortunately, the 'politics of the PFI' has become even more labyrinthine than public planning – with government's agencies (principally the Treasury's Capital Investment Branch, the Department of Health's Private Finance Unit, and the Strategic Health Authority's approval process) creating a huge bureaucracy to add to the 'transactions costs' of dealing with a private 'partner' acting on very different objectives and incentives to the public partner. It is also vital that 'interest rate rules' are consistent regarding payback for both private and public capital – not the case in England now, despite the government still supporting PFIs officially. As often national policies are not 'joined up' with each other.

With PFIs, there is of course a competitive element **before** the preferred private partner (consortium) is chosen by the NHS. This period is governed by EU law, which requires Europe-wide tendering for PFI projects. But this competitive element is lost in the 'no man's land' **after** this choice but **before** the deal is finally signed… the time in which brinkmanship of the utmost sort is generally tried by the private sector.

Overall, there may be limited times when private management and/or public private partnerships are beneficial. But they should be well-tailored to specific needs. PFIs, for example, are not usually– despite the rhetoric –'public/private partnerships'. The latter would require incentives to be aligned across sectors and cultures capable of collaborating, rather than merely contractual clauses of the 'negative' sort.

Summary

While New Labour's first Secretary of State, Frank Dobson, did not favour the private sector (one of the reasons why, like Beckett in opposition in 1995, he was moved in 1999), a new initiative to 'boost' public/private symbiosis was announced soon after his departure, in 2000 (Department of Health, 2000b), **For the Benefit of Patients: A Concordat with the Private and Voluntary Health Provider Sector**. Initiatives mushroomed in the succeeding years. What characterised them all was central **diktat** – national targets, locally enforced through Strategic Health Authorities, for fixed percentages of NHS budgets to be used to buy services from the private sector. This has hastened a crisis for **NHS** capacity, and diminished its capacity to compete in the 'new market' – as well as duplicating 'Treatment Centre' capacity, in some cases, at a time when NHS Boards are being urged to sack doctors as a sign of their credentials in the 'new market'(Nicholson, 2005). In general terms, the private sector is engaged at highly favourable rates, with the 'Payment by Results' scheme applied differently to new private providers (despite the fact that they cover the easier, elective cases and do not have to 'cross subsidise' emergency and specialised care which is (increasingly) inadequately reimbursed.

The biggest idea of them all, for New Labour in its third term especially, has been 'choice and markets'. The next chapter examines what this has meant for the NHS.

Chapter 7

Choice and Markets

Health and Education

The fourth 'idea' to be explored is the biggest of them all. As with the Conservatives in the 1990's, when their 'quasi market' was applied 'across the board' to different public services (health, education, housing and social care) (Bartlett and Le Grand, 1993), the New Labour ideology for public services has come to prioritise 'choice' – prominently in education as well as health. There has been a failure to analyse the similarities and dissimilarities between different policy areas, again, as with the Conservatives in the 1990s. Crudely put, education may be more suitable than health for more radical versions of choice – as ever, we must consider the specific, even technical, uniqueness of each policy area in seeking to apply an idea through the political process (before it becomes a blueprint). Otherwise, a reform quickly has to be re-done – which gives more scope to 'garbage can'-derived policy i.e. the more reviews and decision-points there are, the more scope there is to take the lid off the garbage-can (Greer, 2004).

In both education and health, Old Labour sought to ensure schools and health providers of quality for all through a much more equal society, in which comprehensive education and universal, comprehensive healthcare were not undermined by worse public-sector schools and hospitals in poorer areas. Clearly this vision was not accomplished. And for New Labour, this is seen to be impossible (political economy, again) and even undesirable, if we listen for example to Peter Mandelson – keeping in mind that it was Blair who said, "the New Labour project will be complete when the Labour party has learned to love Peter Mandelson".

Resultingly, New Labour has sought a mechanism by which equal access to providers of high quality in the state sector can be sought, but without assuming geographic equalisation. At the theoretical level, one mechanism is allocation of places by the state. In education, 'bussing' in the United States – in particular, the allocation of poor black children to 'rich' schools – was a means by which equal (in this case, racial) access could be sought, in an unequal society. The guiding ethic was 'equality of opportunity to be unequal' rather than 'equality and opportunity together'. The problem was that this led to a 'flight to private education' as well as being politically unacceptable to middle America. Despite therefore being a policy from the 'land of the free', it is unlikely to appeal to New Labour, involving as it does compulsion of the middle classes through state action. It is however worth noting that, in effect, this is what happens with specialised services, and some emergency services, when the NHS works at its best – people go to the best services in proportion to their need. Unlike with schools, some of the best hospitals are located in poor urban centres.

An alternative to state allocation is consumer choice, which may lead however to selection by provider. The latter is feared by Labour MPs in particular: while grammar schools aided the 'cream' (the brightest, **and** best 'prepared') of the working class, others were 'thrown on the scrap heap at age 11+.' There are two dimensions of 'selection by provider' – transparent use of the criteria by which children (or patients) are eligible for entry; and use of market power by providers to 'cream skim' (and exclude certain categories).

Choice is convenient in fitting both New Labour's belief in markets and – in theory – avoiding 'selection' in education, but the latter is problematic in practice. Schools are chosen by parents on the basis of a variety of 'quality' factors, but children are not barred (officially) on the basis of academic selection. Consumer choice can of course become selection by provider if 'the market does not work'; if over-subscribed schools cannot expand quickly enough (or not without lowering the quality which made them over-subscribed in the first place).

Next, health is actually different from education in key 'market' respects, which is why generic 'public service advisors' to New Labour such as Julian le Grand may well be hasty in proposing generic policy solutions for diverse public services.

Firstly, education is a 'good' for all; healthcare is a 'bad' for an unlucky minority. Education involves a much more homogeneous series of 'products' than health, even allowing for diverse individual and also 'special' needs. Future educational needs can be planned with more stability than in health. Choice has 'transactions costs'; but they are much less than in health. And – for New Labour – the 'status quo' in education is run by local government, with its 'political' and 'parochial' agendas, whereas health is run by agencies under the remit of the central state (or market).

As a result, markets in education make more technical sense as well as being more politically attractive. In education, choice may be a good surrogate for 'bussing'; in health, on the other hand, it may tend more to degenerate into provider selection of consumer rather than vice versa. Indeed, even as New Labour's 'new market' begins seriously in 2006, we see Primary Care Trusts seeking to 'square the circle' of choice and available finance by 'denials of care'. For example, ceilings are put on admissions to hospital (as 'contracts' dominate choice); and patients are denied elective surgery if their Body Mass Index exceeds 30, in various locations across England.

In terms of the analysis of Albert Hirschman (1970), the 'perverse outcomes' to which Hirschman points when markets are used in certain ways seem to apply less to education, although they do apply in some cases. One of the reasons is that 'consumer information' – whether acquired through official data and league tables or in other ways – is more intelligible, more understandable and more 'useable.'

In health, there was 'free choice' of hospital – by GP, communicating with the patient – from 1948 to 1991. It was actually abolished by the Conservatives' internal market in 1991 (when contracts by purchasers restricted the rights of referral by GPs who did not hold their own budget; and GP fundholders in any case often used their own criteria rather than those of patients in exercising choice). This market was based on price competition, to the extent it worked at all. When New Labour took over in 1997, the market was abolished but the 'restriction' of referral was retained. Local services were to be used except in exceptional circumstances ('Out of Area Transfers') rather than the services with which purchasers had 'contracted', as under the Tories' market. Thus New Labour's 'choice' in health is both a 'coming full circle' and incidentally a bureaucratised and limited version of choice. Currently, it is PCTs which 'regulate' (actually manage, often with reference to short-term budgetary needs) GPs' and patients choices of provider – from a menu of either four or five, including at least one 'ISTC' (Independent Sector Treatment Centre). By 2008, it is claimed that choice will be 'free', but this is still being interpreted in the Department of Health as constrained by contracts placed by commissioners, despite appearances to the contrary.

Ironically, planning services at regional level to ensure that specialised and emergency services were coherent could be compatible with choice for 'elective' treatments, in most cases, with 'floors and ceilings' in terms of hospitals' overall viability established by planners. Thus choice would not be limitless, but constraints would be more transparent than those imposed 'by the back door' by the unholy coalition of Monitor and SHAs and PCTs which is currently reducing NHS capacity and making real choice part-fictional and part-trivial.

In practice, choice in the English NHS (with choice meaning something different elsewhere in the UK (Greer 2004)) has to be reconciled with the governments' other policy strands. For example, there is the 'central target' policy. Is a hospital allowed to have lengthened waiting times because it is popular (rather than because it is inefficient or poorly-funded), at least in the medium term? Capacity does not grow overnight – again, expanding hospitals quickly may be even more difficult than for schools. And with costs of expansion 'lumpy' (sometimes with economies of scale; sometimes not), the policy of Payment by Results may be counter-productive: it might be better to allow planners and commissioners to agree variable prices in varying circumstances, even without resorting to a market based on 'price competition.' Economies of scope – benefits from running different services together – may be lost by the choice policy.

Markets More Generally ...

Replacing 'command and control' with 'markets', in public services such as the NHS, often obscures the fact that both lead to – indeed are justified in terms of – a standard 'product'. Post-Fordism in the wider society may necessitate neo-Fordism in the 'welfare product'. Additionally, we can note that the Thatcher reforms required a 'strong state' despite Thatcherite ideology (Gamble, 1981). Likewise, New Labour's repeated attempts to change both structures and incentives, means that the central state will continue to be the key player. Markets in the NHS have to be seen in this context.

We cannot therefore rely on a market distinct enough from politics to fulfil its 'neoclassical' pretensions of allocating efficiently and effectively, and producing equilibrium. If this is so, it is important not to lose the advantages of a planned NHS by comparing 'flawed' planning with an 'idealised' market, (McLachlan and Maynard (Eds), 1982). In 2006, it became apparent that, given the policy of choice, 'new (i.e. modernised) hospitals are necessary; but we no longer know where!' Thus the choice policy came into conflict with the development policy. In particular, the PFI route to developing a new hospital could often be stymied if the local NHS did not know its future income stream, or – worse – its required mix of local and specialist services.

Furthermore, even if a new hospital is needed and authorised, if its local PCT purchasers 'play the market', they as well as the hospital will lose. For if economies of scale are realised through concentrating services in a planned way – rather than 'spreading them thin' over multiple competitors (including private treatment centres) – the savings can be recouped by the whole health economy. Even if the hospital theoretically gains under 'payment by results', it can share the benefits in a cooperative manner with PCTs ('tariff splitting') as long as market incentives do not reduce its ability and willingness so to do.

We see the phoney nature of the NHS market by considering the nature of the 'regulator', Monitor. At least in the privatised utilities, government structured the market and then subsequently a regulator was created. In health, the regulator has been responsible for structuring the market 'on the hoof'. The political dynamics of this in the NHS leave the economic rationale threadbare, as explored below.

Overall, we must remember that firms or providers in a market have a dual role – the 'economic' role of competing (or colluding), assuming it is not a monopoly; and the 'political' role of defending or promoting their interests in the political arena. The latter may be done with the whole industry, or sectionally. Classical economics, involving the theory of 'perfect competition' – and its variant, the pure version of Marxist economics – assumes that firms/providers may not act rationally in terms of long-term interest. Firstly, there is a 'free rider' problem: individual firms will not campaign for the whole industry's health, assuming that someone will else will bear the costs of so doing and that they can reap the benefit. Secondly, under text book assumptions of perfect competition, 'profits are zero' and there are no funds for (for example) building social infrastructure which benefits the firm, unless the latter are supplied by the state. What this means is that, quite apart from collusion within markets, firms and industries which are far-sighted will seek through 'politics' to avoid 'perfect markets' which are both inconvenient and dysfunctional for the long-term.

If the benefits of 'perfect competition' are sought in healthcare, therefore, it requires a regulator single-mindedly focussed upon 're-making markets' when they lapse, specifically as a result of the long-term self-interest of providers; and, resisting perfectly legitimate but countervailing 'planning approaches' (for example, which seek to rationalise bedstock rather than create surplus capacity.) The 1990s internal market foundered on this conundrum (Paton, 1995a). There is already evidence that 'politics' will again lead to the same result this time.

It might then be asked: how do other systems (e.g. in Europe; in parts of the USA) cope with markets in provision? The blunt answer is – their history of over-provision (Paton, 1996b, Ch. 13) allows a transitory market (of maybe a decade or so) as competitive forces, are brought to bear upon a health system which requires re-configuration.

In individual European countries, the more the state steers the healthcare system, primarily in the name of cost-control but in the context of social objectives, as in France in the 1990s, competitive markets will only be affordable in the long run through more generous financing. It is no coincidence that the 'market' initiatives from the European Union which are impacting upon national health systems are associated with, and sometimes causing, greater roles for both private financing and private provision. Rationing within the state sector (either by the available 'envelope' of services or by price, as with co-payments) is currently being accompanied by reform proposals suggesting a greater private/public mix in financing in countries such as Germany and the Netherlands (Paton, 2006c). This replaces the traditional Bismarckian systems which have often had 'separate financing' (mostly private) for the richer (as in Germany and the Netherlands but a state responsibility for 'counting in' the poorer to mostly generous access.

These systems also are now being forced to 'prioritise'. Political economy is the driving force; the European Union's means of both adapting to globalisation and pursuing its own economic and social objectives (Paton *et al*, 2001) is important; and the political distinctiveness of individual countries will shape the means of adaptation.

New Labour and Markets

New Labour's approach is not typical – but neither is it autonomous. It is one means of adapting to the environment of political economy – conditioned by other factors which are significant in conditioning British public policy, such as political structure and the new 'policy culture' described above in Part 2.

Given that New Labour's watch word for the public sector is choice, to some this is a Thatcherite or post-Thatcherite agenda; whereas, to others, it is an attempt to give a social democratic flavour to what would otherwise be market-oriented policies, in an age when both consumer activism and post Fordist political economy render old style public administration obsolete both in practice and in theory.

There is an ongoing tension within New Labour between the state and the market. In terms of the core public services – health and education – this tension is sometimes expressed (at least in the media) in terms of the tension between Blair and Brown. More unites these two in policy terms than divides them (as architects of New Labour, they both have had a fundamentally Atlanticist view of the economy; they both believe in public-private partnerships and particularly the PFI; and they prioritise deregulation over trade union rights). They have however had disagreements about the core public sector. In a nutshell, Blair is excited by even New Right ideas about injecting market forces into the health service, whereas Brown sees the core public services as more of a market-free zone.

Part 2 above sets out how changed international and national political economy is the backdrop to changing policy on the welfare state in Britain i.e. underlying sources of change as opposed to the immediate political conflicts which affect day to day policy. Let us now consider both the theoretical underpinnings to the debate about choice as applied for example to the NHS and how New Labour's policy is being implemented 'on the ground'.

There has been a long standing difference in emphasis between economics and politics – as analysed for example by Albert Hirschman (1970), in *Exit, Voice and Loyalty.* Hirschman was an economist who put the case for political science better than most political scientists, as recognised by Karl Deutsch in his presidential address to the American Political Science Association at the time. In analysing the conditions under which exit, voice (and combinations thereof) have desirable or perverse effects, Hirschman undertook genuine inter-disciplinary work as opposed to merely multi-disciplinary work. There is much that New Labour advisers could have learnt from reading the book more carefully and then seeking to apply – analytically and creatively – the lessons drawn.

Superficially, this has been done. For example Tony Blair's health policy adviser for the year up to 2005, Julian Le Grand (2003), summarised his work over the previous ten years in a book entitled *Motivation, Agency and Public Policy: of Knights and Knaves, Pawns and Queens.* Le Grand genuflects to Hirschman (see page 82 onwards) but does not tackle the breadth and subtlety of Hirschman's argument. Instead he simply documents some problems with using 'voice' as a strategy for improving the performance of public organisations, and then (much more sympathetically) sets out how some of the problems in using 'exit' as a strategy can be overcome. He does the latter by advocating policies for specific public services, in the latter part of the book, based on the quasi-market which seeks to replicate some of the 'text book' advantages of competitive markets. Thus while superficially Le Grand accepts that there is a theoretical and practical choice to be made between voice and exit and that a case can be made for either, his analysis is underpinned by an ideological desire to emphasise exit (as most market-oriented economists do).

Yet if we look at Hirschman, his analysis of **exit, voice**, and then **'a special difficulty in combining exit and voice'**, leads to a chapter entitled, the Elusive Optimal Mix of Exit and Voice. This chapter provides a framework for thinking through, the perverse results which may arise when decline in an organisation arouses primarily from one of exit or voice, yet the organisation is sensitive primarily to the other ie voice or exit. Hirschman considers the 'perverse or pathological cases where an organisation is in effect equipped with a reaction mechanism to which it is not responsive ...'. Simply establishing quasi-markets (even were this possible, and the record of Conservative policy in the 1990s does not suggest it is easy) does not tackle the more subtle points made by Hirschman, and there is no analysis of these types of perverse effects in Le Grand's book.

This is not to suggest that voice is always superior to exit. Clearly this is not so. When we turn to the reality of New Labour's policy, however, we find an obsessive desire with proving post-Thatcherite credentials. New Labour thinks it is accepting the inevitable, and making it desirable; that it is accepting Thatcherite policy but going beyond it. There is a strong view within the citadel of New Labour that anything which smells of statism as opposed to markets, or bureaucracy as opposed to choice, must be treated with deep suspicion. This is the context in which Gordon Brown has been fighting a rearguard action against New Labour stalwarts such as Alan Milburn, Ruth Kelly and David Miliband. It is always Brown who has to do the trimming of the 'new ideas'.

What sort of ideas might we be talking about? Clearly the political fights have been over innovations such as Foundation Hospitals. New Labour-oriented 'think tankers' and advisers such as Ed Mayo (Lea and Mayo, 2002) and Paul Corrigan (health adviser to Blair after 2005) suggested the use of concepts such as the mutual state (where local communities run public services) and the 'public interest company' an allegedly new form of enterprise for public sector service delivery. Even Le Grand (2003), however, is moderately cynical about the underpinning theory (or lack of it) for these trendy concepts. He argues in effect that the incentives they produce are not directed to the ends which are sought. At a political level, in terms of 'signalling left and turning right', it is significant that Mayo's co-author (above) is from the right-wing Institute of Directors.

In effect the think tankers and policy advisers have come up with **soundbites** which, when examined, present old ideas – not much different from the voluntary hospitals and autonomous 'not for profit' organisations operating throughout the Bismarckian health systems of Europe and the traditional, fast shrinking, non profit sector of the United States since the 1950s. In other words, these are the institutions which are obsolete in a tightly managed or 'market' world.

There are 'liberal' (ie capitalist) or Rightist think tanks – such as Reform and Civitas, more recently, and the best known from the 1980s and 1990s (the Centre for Policy Studies, the Institute of Economic Affairs Health Unit; and the Adam Smith Institute) – which present European healthcare systems such as Germany's as the future rather than the past. This is doubly ironical. For the Right identifies these countries as schlerotic and requiring an injection of Anglo-American market forces in both economy and welfare sectors. So why the eulogies for their health systems – which are in any case being transformed – unless for the ideological purpose of denigrating statist systems. Additionally the direct taxation for health benefits in such economies is higher than in the UK. The **real** agenda is privatisation, which would produce very different results in England from the socialised healthcare systems of France and Germany. The question is therefore: what is New Labour doing by flirting with such analysis, at the very least being influenced by it?

Economics tends to stress 'exit'; and political science and sociology tend to stress 'voice' i.e. collective and non market solutions to poor performance. What sort of combinations of exit and voice might we best apply to the core public sector in Britain today? That is the challenge for policy analysis. The political question is, how do we explain the shape of New Labour's policy? For it has not proceeded from neutral policy analysis.

Fist Over Hand – The New Market and Choice in the English NHS

As England (unlike the rest of the UK) retreads the market route in health policy, it is worth asking two questions. Firstly, is the government right that the 'new market' (as it refuses to call it, except in private seminars) is fundamentally different from the 1990s' internal market which New Labour allegedly abolished in 1997? Secondly, given that the new market is clearly not characterised by the invisible hand, should we characterise it as steered 'economically' by a visible (facilitating) hand, on the one hand, or managed 'politically', by a fist which would like to remain invisible in order to maintain its power? It is useful to invoke Hirschman (1970) as a stimulus to critical reflection, upon how 'exit', 'voice' and particular combinations of 'exit' and 'voice', may produce perverse outcomes.

The New Market

In a nutshell, the new NHS market is used allegedly to promote competition on the basis of quality not price. The old 1990s internal market is characterised by New Labour as having promoted price competition. This in turn supposedly led to a stress on 'widgets' – quantity, but only at the margin, in order to get extra deals, rather than quality, and also led to corner-cutting. There is evidence (Propper et al, 2004) that the less successful competitor Trusts in the old market exhibited worse clinical outcomes (presumably as they cut costs to compete). There is also evidence that competition was wasteful and counter-productive on the occasions when it genuinely occurred, with purchasers moving contracts without evidence of benefit (Paton et al, 1998). Yet there is also evidence that, in general, competition did not occur (except as a new name for the type of reconfiguration of services which had always happened), as the excess capacity to make it possible was forbidden by the government – running a Janus-faced policy. (Paton, 1995a) In the end, the old market was abolished long before Labour made its 1997 promise to abolish it…except for the purchaser/provider split which Labour did not abolish but deepened (Paton, 1999a). New Labour's big idea, not original but important, was clinical governance and quality. The question now is how this is compatible with the new market.

The new market's analytics are contained in the 'payment by results' policy (PBR), which eschews price competition by setting a national tariff (with regional adjustments) at national average cost for clinical treatments grouped into Healthcare Resource Groups (HRGs.) This has an equivocal message for quality. Where services at higher cost/price and quality are desired by purchasers (commissioners), this is prohibited: the tariff is the tariff is the tariff (except when it is not – i.e. when political intervention alters its effect). This is a dangerous situation when the tariff may be plain wrong, and there is evidence that some specialised services are wrongly costed/priced (the same, since price is set at average cost). As a result, Trusts – especially Foundation Trusts, with marginally more freedom – may disinvest in needed services: if this happens by market decision rather than in a strategic framework or as part of a plan, then holes may appear in the NHS menu of services.

What the new market seeks is 'the maximum quality compatible with the price set by the tariff'. If provider Trusts are in a competitive local or regional market and 'need the business', then the complementary policy of patient choice will allegedly force them to cut costs (if they need to) to tariff, or below, and maximise quality to the extent necessary to attract patients.

If they want to cross-subsidise services which the tariff deems expensive, Trusts will have to cut costs below tariff for other services. Thus there will be a tension between cutting costs and promoting quality – which, if actors are rational, will be resolved by factors such as the degree of 'consumerism' in the local population. Where this is less (i.e. where 'the public wants what the public gets'), trusts will get away with murder, hopefully not literally. And if they do not want to cross-subsidise (e.g. to protect specialised services where the tariff is arguably wrong), then the danger of omission will arise as argued above.

History is repeating itself from the 1990s in one major way. Foundation Trusts are being fed the rhetoric of self-determination – that they may decide their service mix, within limits decided in practice by 'the economic regulator', Monitor. Thus the whole of the NHS may be less than the sum of its parts, as just argued. But more than this: to run a market means excess capacity, so that providers can quickly react to demand (given that hospital services are not bananas or umbrellas – they take time to develop). In the language of transactional economics, there is a problem with asset specificity.

Yet, as in the 1990s, hospitals are, as we speak, being 'stripped out', to make them lean and mean market machines (the real agenda for Foundation Trusts… forget the hypocrisy about stakeholding). So where will the capacity come from? The government would argue, "from the Independent Sector Treatment Centres (ISTCs) and other market entrants" (mostly at the point of the government's gun rather than commissioner choice). The problem is that the new competitors can only be afforded by the said 'stripping out' in the traditional NHS. To complain of this is not to be sentimental, or to exhibit Blair's dreaded symptom, that of being the "forces of conservatism". What it means is that there is no genuine competition, but a rigged market.

As the cream is skimmed by ISTCs and others, fixed costs left in the NHS hospitals (even after 'stripping out') cannot easily be spread over the more difficult and specialised services, plus the flood of emergencies, which remain within tariff for these services. When another factor occurs, we have the 'double whammy': already, the government is cutting the tariff, service by service, to add to existing 'efficiency savings', a neologistic misnomer for arbitrary economies. As a result, good hospitals will be 'slashed and burned' and good services will be lost. The tariff for certain categories of specialised services, in particular, is too crude to account for the most complex case-mixes. And it is deliberate policy to reduce 'price per HRG' over time – overtly to put pressure upon hospitals' costs but surreptitiously to 'square the circle' of need or demand and available resources. To give an example of the latter: for 2006-7, emergency 'over performance' (i.e. demand at the hospital portals which commissioners or GPs have been unable to control) are to be reimbursed at 'half-tariff only.'

Even worse: some hospitals are in financial deficit not through inefficiency but through inadequate reimbursement for the workload they cannot control. In general, Strategic Health Authorities (SHAs) – the 'internal NHS regulators' – insist they do this work, thus de facto encouraging Primary Care Trust purchasers (PCTs) to 'game the system'. And absurdly, SHAs then seek to broker money to the hospitals in deficit through 'top slicing' from the PCTs (i.e. cutting their budget) – which the PCTs promptly pass on to the hospitals in reduced income. Whether this is described as 'politics' or the Gods making mad those whom they wish to destroy, it is certainly not a transparently-regulated market.

To this bilious mix, let us fold in consumerism. Which providers will (increasingly well-informed) consumers find attractive – those being cut to the bone, with lengths of stay slashed and 'no frills' service, on the one hand, or gerrymandered new market entrants? It seems obvious that they'll choose the latter (which are good at marketing themselves but with unproven clinical quality) but if we are to have a market, we have to at least get the NHS to the starting-line.

The Political Fist

The new NHS market is clearly not a competitive market guided by Adam Smith's invisible hand. This need not be a criticism. Just as some text-book idealists had aspirations for a 'quasi-market' in the 1990s, the new market might be defended as an attempt, in a different way, to combine 'animal spirits' and altruism.

The trouble with the old 1990s version was that government could not make up its mind if its 'regulation' (then internal regulation, by government and its minions in the Regions of the NHS) was intended to dampen down market forces (good old-fashioned political management) or to stimulate them (to put the market into 'quasi', as it were). This led to the absurdity of hospitals being ordered to compete and collaborate at the same time, even at the level of individual specialties.

Now, the rhetoric is marginally more sophisticated. We are told that, in mature 'industrial' markets, both competition and collaboration occur – and that market actors can gradually sort out for themselves where and when they do each (improving on the old market's political confusion, in which action was in response to temporary political orders, each incompatible with the last). Good so far. But can 'they' keep the politics out? A few straws in the wind suggest that a politics-free zone is like Gandhi's take on Western civilisation – a good idea, but it'll never happen.

Le Grand (2003) has suggested that altruism and self-interest (co-existing within key NHS actors as well as differently distributed across different groups such as doctors and managers) may both be moulded into a market framework to benefit a (presumably altruistically-defined) NHS. The problem is that this ticklishly difficult combination assumes that 'politics' sets up the perfect model and then benignly withdraws. I contend, however, that the invisible fist – which uses fragments of economic logic as a figleaf for 'informal' but determinant political and bureaucratic power – is the basis for decision-making as to (provider) service reconfiguration and (purchaser/commissioner) behaviour – just as in the 1990s. The main difference now is also political rather than economic: New Labour (unlike the Conservative Secretary of State for Health who designed the 1990s reforms, Kenneth Clarke) believes its own rhetoric. This may leave idealists like Le Grand somewhat disillusioned when they interact with political power. Le Grand was surprised in the mid-1990s when he apprised the reality of 'market management' (i.e. Regional political intervention acting with national blessing) to protect services which were falling through the market's cracks (Conversation with Author, Keele University, 1994). As his own market prescriptions today are merged into a cocktail of contradictory policy prescriptions leaving a confused patient (the NHS) distinctly queasy, he may be experiencing a similar frisson.

Today, 'politics' is already shaping the English NHS according to an agenda very different from that eulogised by the marketeers. Firstly, the external and internal regulators – i.e. Monitor and the Strategic Health Authorities (SHAs) respectively – struggle to help each other. Monitor gets 'the books balanced' (for most hospitals, not just Foundation Trusts, on the grounds that Monitor is the agency charged with developing NHS Trusts into Foundation Trusts). Monitor seeks financial viability on an individual Trust basis, rather than for wider health economies as part of a broader strategy – which makes for fragmented service planning. The SHA, in turn, loses some direct influence, but of the sort it found awkward in the first place – i.e. strategically managing the area for which it was responsible, rather than the easier task of 'performance monitoring' the Trusts and PCTs in that area. And the SHA can hide behind Monitor's skirts in enforcing political and personnel changes it wishes to make in Trusts, the pretext for which has hitherto been elusive.

Secondly, Monitor, by seizing centre stage and political power as well as 'economic regulation', will then have to manage the 'market', not just regulate it. It was extraordinary naivety, as well as amnesia, which left **overall** system regulation off the agenda, as New Labour rushed to market. SHAs, as all Trusts gradually become Foundations (i.e. formally external to the NHS 'lines of control' and therefore responsible to the external regulator, Monitor, rather than to the SHA), will yield to Monitor over time. It was intended that SHAs, themselves merging into pale replicas of the old English Regions, would also yield interventionary powers to the new 'strategic' Primary Care Trusts (PCTs), post-2006. However, in 2006, the Secretary of State for Health backtracked on plans for radical as opposed to incremental mergers of PCTs – in reaction to backbench MPs and the Parliamentary (House of Commons) Health Select Committee, given the reduced parliamentary majority for the governing party. (Sir Nigel Crisp, the NHS Chief Executive and also Permanent Secretary to the Department of Health was forced to resign on March 7th, 2006, in part because he 'carried the can' for a Ministerial policy which now embarrassed Ministers.) Backbench MPs – as discussed in Part 2 – tend to see 'their' local PCTs as symbols of their influence – in US terms, 'the bacon which they have brought home to their districts.' It is, however, symbolic and indeed indigestible bacon, as the most notable role for local PCTs has been to seek to lengthen local waiting-times for operations in order to postpone financial crisis.

The idea of larger, 'strategic' PCTs was that they would be relieved of direct commissioning in order to promote 'Practice-Based Commissioning' (PBC) which devolves commissioning to groups of GPs (borrowing from the 1990s policy of GP fund-holding). The PCTs are still intended to manage 'non-contestable services' (such as Accident and Emergency networks and specialist services). Yet even larger PCTs are too small-scale to do this, and in any case their record in this regard is poor in the extreme. What is the biggest irony of all is that the smaller PCTs are being reinvented, as GP practices (charged with running PBC) merge for commissioning: purposes into small-area PCTs in all but name. As ever, 'efficiency' becomes management cost.

The newly-merged 'strategic' PCTs are to set increasingly local standards, which is a major conflict-of-interest as they hold the purse strings and have the power to pressurize hospitals but not the responsibility to provide effective services. According to 'Commissioning a Patient-led NHS' (Department of Health, 2005), Primary Care Trusts were to have been stripped of their provider function. This made sense if knavery rather than knightly behaviour (in Le Grand's (2003) terms) were considered to rule – i.e. there was a conflict-of-interest between commissioning and provision. The trouble is that knavery did not prevail as a matter of course but was promoted (as in the 1990s, the culture of which was still lingering) by a constant stress upon markets and contracts rather than trust and cooperation.

Given the fact that pro-market health advisers had Prime Minster Blair's ear (and that of the Secretaries of State for Health under New Labour after Frank Dobson was replaced by Alan Milburn in 1999), 'cooperation' within local health economies (despite being encouraged officially) was mistrusted in reality (for example, former Ministerial and Prime Ministerial health adviser Simon Stevens (2005) suggested that 'integrated health economies' would involve collusion by doctors.) This 'smoke and mirrors' puts local health executives in an impossible position: when they cooperate, they fall foul of deliberately-designed market incentives; and when they follow those incentives, they are blamed and even treated as scapegoats by the 'meso-level political managers' at the SHA for not cooperating.

And as a result of real as opposed to phoney cooperation being dismissed as collusion, hospital Trusts were generally not to be allowed to be the basis for, or even a partner in, vertically-integrated services (replicating HMOs), despite Kaiser Permanente in California impressing Ministers and despite this being a classic example of how to create a mature 'industrial market' rather than a naïve NHS 'banana market'.

Finally, good old fashioned command and control – or more accurately 'kiss up; kick down', in the vernacular used in US government – has had a premature obituary. As we have seen, Secretary of State for Health Alan Milburn announced its death in 2002, in order to deny that the NHS after his 2002 reforms would be 'Stalinist'. His successor Secretaries of State have continued to 'kick down', expecting the meso-level bureaucrats in the NHS to be political fixers rather than 'neutral' regulators.

The visible hand is intended to be the new PCT-as-standard setter and regulator of commissioning. But the invisible fist is what rationalises the four incompatible policy streams to have emerged from the 'garbage can' of recent health policy and still extant in various degrees. The four are: firstly, the old market, based on purchaser contracting; secondly, the 'third way' of local 'collaboration' (but at the point of a gun, as the collaborators fight like ferrets in a sack); thirdly, neo-'command and control', based on various targets promulgated down seriously 'un-joined up' vertical silos from the Department of Health; and fourthly, the new market of patient choice underpinned shakily by 'Payment By Results'.

Choice and Hirschman

Albert Hirschman's (1970) classic little book was in essence an attempt by a renowned economist to do genuinely inter-disciplinary work between economics and politics, in language both elegant and accessible. He sought to explore when 'exit' and 'voice' – and particular combinations thereof – would have benign and perverse outcomes in different industrial, organisational and political settings. The 'choice debate' in the English NHS has equated 'market choice' with 'exit' from providers. The resulting analysis, however, has omitted some key considerations.

Firstly, competition – exit – may be intended (as Le Grand admits) to send a signal to sub-standard providers to help them improve. Yet it may work too quickly or too abruptly and close them down (or debilitate them, if closure is politically impossible). This is a real danger in the NHS, where the tariff under Payment-by-Results will (from 2006) cover the total cost/price of Trust services. 'A fool learns from his own mistakes; a wise man learns from those of others'. We had the chance to do the latter; but now others, abroad, will have a good case study of what not to do. The Department of Health thinks it has learned from other European, North American and Australian systems of prospective reimbursement, but in fact has implemented on a scale which they (wisely) did not (as with the rash decision to let the tariff cover capital as well as revenue). This rash decision means that, in Hirschman's terms, 'exit' by consumers and loss of full tariff may cripple a hospital too quickly to allow it to respond to market signalling. The effect may be enhanced if the hospital is undergoing a large Private Finance Initiatives (PFI) i.e. using a private partner to finance development in order to keep government borrowing down. Market repayment rate to the private sector is about double that of the NHS internal 'capital charge', and loss of income at 'full tariff' may send the hospital into crisis rather than give it a useful signal.

Secondly, competition can comfort monopoly. If the more demanding consumers go elsewhere, Trusts can have a quieter life, as long as their market contains enough uncompetitive elements and they retain enough services to be viable at all. If Trusts seek 'break-even' rather than surplus – as they do – this may be particularly compelling.

Thirdly, competition may be a zero-sum game. This was a compelling lesson from the old NHS market. As in the old market, patients may move from Provider X to Y while simultaneously patients move from Y to X – to no discernible benefit in either health outcomes or patient satisfaction (indeed, choice may make you miserable). What is more, commissioners are actually only purchasers: that is, they negotiate deals rather than craft new services cooperatively. And even that only occurs if we're lucky: many are retrospective 'contract-breakers' who agree 'service level agreements' with providers as part of the so-called NHS budgetary process, and then seek to renege on these at the end of the financial year.

Local commissioners will have little ability to be 'market makers', despite the glib rhetoric. It is not just a question of 'further development for commissioners', the tired (and arguably self-serving) old mantra of many health analysts and consultants who are too ingenuous about each cycle of health reform: it is instead a question of how patient choice will be reconciled with purchaser choice. The two together create local conflicts which are already summoning the invisible fist rather than the transparent regulatory hand. Political amnesia (which forgets even the last decade) combined with academic naivety is a dangerous thing.

Fourthly, price and quality have different elasticities. Those who would tolerate price rises may exit at the drop of a hat due to a small decline in quality. In the NHS consumers do not pay (at the point of use), but they may exit quickly, to the private sector, and may fail to return even if the private sector's quality also declines (since they have invested both economically and psychologically in the change). Thus, the political legitimacy of the NHS – and the economic viability, as willingness to pay taxes for unused services falls – may decline.

This does not mean that 'voice' has been effective in the NHS Le Grand is right that it has **not**. Indeed initiatives to increase consumer or citizen 'voice' (such as 'Patient and Public Involvement' since 2002) have been at best marginal and at worst diversionary. But Hirschman's key insights are around perverse outcomes associated with different combinations of voice and exit in different circumstances. For example, if some 'exit' (from a provider) leaving only those who refuse to exit out of loyalty, the latter may be the wrong constituency to promote change or innovation. As in education, 'sink hospitals' serving those who do not exit through commuting may stagger on – because they have to – just as 'sink schools' are left behind by the brave new world of Blairite 'choice.'

More rigorous examination of 'choice and voice' is required if the latest NHS reforms in England are not to end up in the dustbin of history, as with the reforms in the 1990s. Secondly, the centralist political culture of the NHS is deeply-entrenched, and buttressed by both structural aspects of the British political system and now (ironically) the 'post-modern' style of policy-making which makes the 'eye-catching central initiative' both ephemeral and yet endemic. In this environment, reconciling a 'devolved market' with public accountability for a centrally-funded service may be to enter the territory of the oxymoron.

In the 1990s, 'managed competition' had the choice of becoming either management or market. The Conservative Government reluctantly chose the former. New Labour boasts that "the main difference between the Tory reforms in the 1990s and us is that they 'bottled out' (meaning that they lost their nerve) (Paul Corrigan made this claim in 2003 when Special Advisor to the Health Secretary.) New Labour Ministers are desperate to show that there is a 'third way' (although they have dropped that Clintonesque phrase); that 'regulated competition' in a public service is the answer.

Whether or not they 'bottle out', I believe they are wrong. Reconciling the conflicting policy strands in today's English NHS means either the victory of public planning or the decline of the NHS as a public service. The trouble is that, in the structure and culture of the English NHS today, public planning has to be done by the backdoor, enforced by the invisible fist. It therefore lacks both consistency and legitimacy. It need not be so. The government could admit that 'commissioning' is a fudge, with service planning and 'purchasing' merged to the detriment of the former, and institute effective service planning. Planning is a frightening word for New Labour, with its New Right connections, but service planning at regional level can relieve the centre of its need to control so obsessively. The trouble is that Regional Health Authorities were abolished by the Conservatives in 1996, to be replaced by more 'on message' Regional Offices, in turn abolished by Labour in 2001. The cultural question is, can New Labour give up its 'control-freak' tendency?

Rationalising the Irrational

The last two chapters have explored some (not all) of the ideas which have characterised New Labour's stewardship of the NHS. These themes and the political agency which has both produced them and sought to act on them should like all ideas be understood in their structural and cultural context. Part 2 of this book has set out the stages of New Labour's ongoing NHS reform. The 'elephant in the room' is of course the previous Conservative government's 'internal market' reforms. New Labour inherited – and accepted – the structures bequeathed by these reforms, even in the early years (1997-1999) when it (partially) rejected the culture they had engendered.

Yet, as BP, McKinsey and other private sector actors have indicated, 'structure is strategy'. While the stages of policy listed in Part 2 did indeed emerge piecemeal from the 'garbage can', they were absorbed by a structural and cultural context which mobilised bias as to what they became. In a nutshell, a 'bias to the market' grew; and the rhetoric of (and institutional tinkering geared towards) 'devolution' also grew.

At one level, this was making a virtue of necessity (We've got pluralist disaggregation, in the NHS, so we might as well pretend it was intended). Also, the ideas outlined in Part 3 of the book were part–rationality, part-predilection, part–inheritance and part–convenience. For example, shifting resources out of hospital ('hospital bad/primary care good') may be rational ('who wants to stay in hospital too long and catch MRSA?'). It genuflects to the old 'community' tradition (which is about all that New Labour Ministers have left of their founding beliefs); it gels with the structures inherited (a multiplicity of 'primary care authorities' which pursue their own localist agendas, often irrespective of system-wide effects); and it legitimises severe cost-reductions made in hospitals for short-termist, fiscal reasons rather than as part of strategy.

Overall however, to the extent that rationalisation is occurring – and to the extent that strategy is 'emergent' (ie. rationalising, not causing, what is happening) – it is too difficult for New Labour to make the case for an integrated, publicly-provided NHS. It is too difficult ideologically (Blairism is 'in blood stepp'd in so far ...'); it is too difficult politically (there are too many micro-interests, created by cycles of reform, to be offended); it is too difficult organisationally (New Labour has 're-dis-organised' so often that it cannot, paradoxically, undertake the ultimate 're-form' of abolishing a whole swathe of ill thought-out reforms); and it is too difficult managerially.

It is too difficult managerially because that would mean creative attainment of plural goals (integrated services; efficiency; quality) through effective leadership of altruistically – motivated organisations. Far easier (it seems) to set market forces to divide and rule. Which brings us back to culture: that is the culture which any 'new reform' would have to deal with.

None of this is to deny the need for 'productivity', 'shorter length of stay' (if community services are integrated with hospital strategy), 'better procurement' and all the desiderata endlessly recycled at great profit to management consultants (Leys, 1999). It is simply to remind ourselves that the rationale for 'the market' is at root political rather than based upon evaluation of health reform whether domestic or international. Interestingly, the divergent paths of the four UK NHSs, post-devolution may eventually shed some light on whether 'there is no alternative' to the English/Blairite route-map.

Chapter 8

The State of New Labour's Healthcare State

The Politics of the 'Third Way'

Health policy in England – in the sense of 'high politics' i.e. political decisions as to the shape of the health system – is driven primarily by ideological factors, rather than technical factors aimed at increasing the cost-effectiveness of public expenditure and/or improving quality (Paton, 2005). As a result, initiatives geared to the latter ends (of which there are many worthy ones) have to be implemented often in a roundabout way, through institutions which are less than fit for purpose, creating complexity in implementation. Reconciling ideologically-motivated yet piecemeal 'chunks' of policy – including Foundation Trusts and various versions of the 'new internal market' – is problematical, not just because of the opportunity cost of the effort but because different chunks of policy are based in different incentive systems and even different values. The challenge for the future is to simplify and synthesise policy on the basis of adequate consensus between the state, the medical profession and the public (Salter, 1998; Klein, 2000)

New Labour's rhetoric rejects the 'direct provision' state for the regulatory state (Jessop, 2002). Yet the reality is often greater centralization – not because the 'new devolution' based on 'shifting the balance of power' (Department of Health, 2001) is too timid, but because it is born in a looking-glass world. Strategic Health Authorities and (especially) Primary Care Trusts have responsibility, not power. The new arrangements in the NHS mean that the key capital and planning decisions (such as the creation of new hospitals, especially under the PFI) are centralized fair square to the Department of Health, in the absence of Regions. The challenge for the future here is to achieve an appropriate mix between devolution and centralism which is transparent, stable and designed around health policy functions rather than piecemeal political initiatives.

From 1948 to 1991 the NHS was the antithesis of 'command and control'. Alongside traditional public administration sat medical networks (both benign and otherwise). What Mrs. Thatcher hoped to get from her internal market was a means of control to ensure that her commands – or, more charitably, central priorities – were implemented. What New Labour has been about in its first five years is deepening the control in pursuit of an (admirably) wider set of central priorities, putting quality and

– to an extent – equality on the agenda alongside bean-counting (Paton, 1999). The Third Way, in British health policy, to the extent it was anything, was an alternative to both command and control (the first way) and then the internal market (the second way), mirroring the economy-wide Third Way following 'old-style social democracy' (first way) then Thatcherism (second way). But since the characterization of 1948-1991 in the NHS by New Labour was wrong, that leaves the Third Way as misleading rhetoric – and its co-existence with the reality of command-and-control in the NHS since early in New Labour's first term has been uneasy, to say the least.

Exworthy and Halford (1999) are right to put both the new managerialism and quasi-markets in context, and to point to quasi-markets, quasi-hierarchies and quasi-networks. A hierarchy which does not provide the basis for 'commanding' the doctors is 'quasi' at best. Indeed the quasi-market and the 'networks' approach (which developed within the bosom of the internal market (Flynn, 1992), rather than from the rhetoric of the Third Way, in any case) were both attempts to render the medical profession corporately responsible. Alongside creating consistency, coherence and parsimony from the plethora of 'new institutions' in and over the NHS, this remains the biggest challenge – to which clinical governance, appraisal, re-validation and the new consultant contract will, it is hoped, make a big contribution.

This is less a Third Way than the unfinished business of the Griffiths reforms of 1983 onwards, from which the internal market was a huge distraction (which incidentally destroyed a lot of the 'meso' institutions required for the strategic planning of public health services.) Ironically, Labour's stance around 1992 was a sensible one – accepting the Griffiths legacy, while rejecting the internal market... yet seeking a framework for performance management which rewarded successful organizations, incorporated clinical assessment and did so in the context of unified (what would now be called) 'local health economies' and appropriate regional planning (The Labour Party, 1992). Indeed, to be fair, many of New Labour's keynote 'quality' and even 'performance incentive' initiatives were present in embryo in the policy papers developed earlier (see also The Labour Party, 1995).

The complication now is the policy and institutional inheritance, which has created a 'mobilisation of bias' in policy-making towards a new ideological approach. Here the future challenge is to separate the wheat from the chaff in policies and structures. New Labour both inherited the 'Thatcher reforms' to the NHS's structure and culture and also promulgated (especially from 2001 onwards) its own 'mixed economy' agenda for the NHS (Milburn, 2002). Paradoxically, this plethora of systems and initiatives is obstructing genuine devolution in the NHS.

We find an obsession with denying 'Stalinism' ("the...unprecedented ideological onslaught from the Right...determined to bring down what they now freely describe as a 'Stalinist' creation) (Milburn, 2002.) Later in the same speech, we find reference to the "middle ground between state-run public and shareholder-led private structures... (embraced by)...both the Right...and the Left – through the Co-operative Movement." Is this the same Right which wishes to bring down the NHS, or a different one? If the latter, what is the basis for ascribing the difference? If the former, is it really better to get into bed, ideologically speaking, with the wreckers, rather than to deny the charge of Stalinism more radically? And was this always New Labour's big idea?

'Targets and Standards': Are Standards a Practical Third Way?

It is no exaggeration to say that clinical governance was the 'big idea' of New Labour's first term. Many components of clinical governance (such as clinical audit) were not new, but the incoming government in 1997 wished to signal a new emphasis to the NHS. In opposition, Labour had criticised the Conservatives' internal market in the NHS between 1991 and the mid-1990s (Paton et al, 1998), arguing that it emphasized bean counting rather than quality. Indeed later, rather alarming work suggested that "the relationship between competition and quality appears to be negative" : hospitals located in more competitive areas during the internal market had higher death rates for certain conditions, after adjusting for other explanations. (Propper et al, 2003) It was against the backdrop of suspicion of the internal market that Labour's focus upon clinical governance was to be buttressed by collaboration within 'health economies' rather than competition.

Clearly this is still an important strand of policy, which has evolved in the direction of the new **standards** for healthcare. The seven 'core' and 'developmental' standards emphasize quality, safety and the need to provide integrated care along the patient 'pathway' ie. integrated case across organisational boundaries, necessitating cooperation between providers – and between 'commissioners' and providers. Clinical networks, which were arguably a 'bottom up' response to the fragmentation of 'top down' national policy in the form of the former internal market, are an important part of this picture. The Healthcare Commission (HCC), which is responsible for assessing Trusts against the standards, in an annual 'health check', has furthermore made some criticisms of how **targets** have hitherto been used in the NHS. The HCC has intended that the national system of performance assessment, which succeeded star ratings in 2006, will emphasize 'qualitative' factors to a greater extent.

Quantitative targets are not all bad – far from it – even including the headline 'political' targets. Focusing on waiting times for consultations and treatments (and in A and E), have been responsible for huge improvements in performance – for patients, not just in order to 'tick the box' for the Strategic Health Authority (SHA) and the Department of Health. Targets at their best are based upon measures of performance which relate to clinical quality and patients' experience. Targets without incentives and/or sanctions, moreover, might not have the desired effect. The challenge is to improve both individual targets and the basket of targets which is used to measure the overall performance of a Trust. There is academic debate about whether performance measures should be aggregated in this way, but the motivating nature of 'three star status' or equivalent is very powerful – not just at Board and Executive level within Trusts but throughout the whole organisation. Even cynics about targets should remember that they are like the nuclear bomb: in the information age of better informed service users, they cannot be 'un-invented.'

The problem arises when targets are set inappropriately or policed unimaginatively. One does not need to be an economist to know that extra investment has alternative uses – and a challenge for government is to be more analytical in how politicians and Department of Health executives 'trade off' different targets, all of which have implications for the use of resources (money, and the time of management, clinicians and indeed all staff.) For example: should the A and E 'four hour target' have been set to 98%, lower or higher – and what are the alternative uses of resources?

Politicians, think-tanks and academics and NHS staff all live in different worlds, to some extent, and they will always have different ways of looking at things. Sustainable improvements have emerged from 'tough targets', as well as – sometimes – unintended outcomes. Indeed, even the latter (eg clinicians claiming that perverse prioritisation occurs) are sometimes overblown – in that, at its best, a 'target culture' may improve performance, such as waiting times, for everyone.

But that does not mean there should not be more consensus around a shared agenda than at present. Politicians also have a responsibility to govern (and 'police') sensitively. If targets are set by the government to aid spin geared to 'dishing the opposition' and then presented to the Department of Health's management team as the 'be-all and end-all', then in all likelihood a 'chain of command' will lead to the various 'sorcerer's apprentices' throughout the system running amok, as in Disney's Fantasia! The internal regulatory agencies of the NHS such as SHAs will be forced to play numbers games, crowding out the time they have for challenges such as reconfiguring health services.

The real problem with today's NHS policy is not targets per se, but the excessive overload of 'initiatives' which grow into full-blown radical policy changes. This is not a gripe about change from what the Prime Minister called 'the forces of conservatism.' It is an observation that there are currently four different, conflicting streams of policy being used to steer the NHS.

One is the '1990s' purchaser/provider split, renamed but alive and unwell after Shifting the Balance of Power. The second is the target approach. The third is the 'new market' of patient choice and payment by results. And the fourth is 'collaboration'. The second and third are really alternatives (the former based on hierarchy; the latter based on competition), although they may co-exist if handled sensitively. More importantly however, the first makes the fourth very difficult.

It would be better if real patient choice for 'electives' coexisted with cooperative health economies, realising the benefits of networks and a reconciliation of planning and commissioning at a higher level. Then targets and standards could be shared properly, and collaboratively, across the different parts of the NHS.

Revisiting 'The New Regulatory State?'

The idea of the new regulation is that the state is 'hollowed out' – with regulation replacing provision in a welfare state which mirrors the wider 'post Fordist' economy.

(Burrows and Loader, 1994). This may involve both devolution and centralisation from previous sources of both authority and provision.

Devolution was the soundbite around which Shifting the Balance of Power was framed. Ideologically, devolution provides a response to the charge of Stalinism. Practically, it allows Primary Care Trusts to be packaged as devolution, when they were already on the agenda – being New Labour's means of absorbing (and arguably extending) GP fundholding and also the Total Purchasing arrangements at the fag-end of the Tory years. This absorption was a means of keeping the 1997 promise of NHS 'reintegration without re-organisation.' Yet it stored up trouble which the Department of Health sought (only partially) to address in 2005.

Inspection is the quid-pro-quo of devolution. One should really talk of regulation via performance indicators and inspection, with performance management to be carried out by Strategic Health Authorities (SHAs) in the absence of a Regional tier.

The problem here is that, given the perverse incentives created by the deepened purchaser/provider split between NHS Trusts and Primary Care Trusts respectively, local health economies (covering populations of around half a million or less) have no integrating mechanism other than goodwill or mutual dependence in meeting targets. SHAs tend to monitor performance rather than manage it: that is, they receive Local Delivery Plans from Trusts, but have no ability to align funding flows with service plans. The SHA should be the planner of last resort, but this is rendered difficult by deliberately creating disaggregation under the banner of devolution. In other words the political and ideological agenda – presenting PCTs (in fact the semi-legitimate offspring of the Conservative reforms) as the source of devolution in the NHS – clashes with the analytical policy agenda of achieving objectives and targets effectively and efficiently. Service priorities and funding streams are not aligned.

Regulation can refer to economic regulation (of structures, such as the form of markets; institutions, such as health care providers; and/or processes, such as the PFI, 'foundation Trusts' et al) or to standard-setting via outcomes, primarily quality and equality in clinical and other services. At first, it seemed that New Labour, in abolishing the internal market, would be replacing the former with the latter. Now since New Labour has re-invented the market, it will require both. A practical question therefore arises: should regulation be global, covering all aspects together or will different agencies tackle their own domains, from the structure of the market through the provision of adequate resources to the inspection of quality.

If regulation is global, the distinction between policy, regulation and provision may break down in practice. That is, if inspection covers inter alia quality of services, the need for resources and appropriate relationships between providers, it becomes policy – and government will not want that contracted out.

The work-remit for the National Institute for Clinical Excellence (NICE), for example, is set by the government. The Bank of England, it could be argued, also has its central objective (the inflation rate) set by the government, which is the criterion to be used in setting interest-rates. But NICE is more circumscribed: it is not given a resource envelope and then told to 'get on and do the QALYs' (in order to meet the central objective of maximizing health gain within available resources); it makes piecemeal decisions.

If regulation overall is more piecemeal, two important things may happen: firstly, regulation may be shared between 'genuine' regulators (i.e. agencies with autonomy outside the governmental chain of command) and line agencies within the DoH or NHS (e.g. StHAs); and, secondly, different regulators may prioritise differently when 'feeding back' to providers; indeed, may individually 'command' such that the total sum of commands is internally contradictory or 'not do-able' in the here and now. This is of course the current state-of-affairs, which I will happily illustrate wearing the hat of a large acute Trust Chairman, whose Trust is regularly visited by branches of the NHS, often stipulating different priorities.

Now, let us consider 'autonomy' on the one hand and health service targets on the other hand. It is clear that the 'new devolution' does not involve the centre relinquishing its role in setting targets, but refers instead to qualified operational freedoms. Whether this is autonomy or a radical exercise of power by the centre is a moot point.

More practically, there is a real debate to be had about whether the centre should specify generic outcomes (e.g. health of populations) or specific targets, and indeed whether politicians should yield to an 'NHS Board' in setting (definitely) the latter and (possibly) the former. The King's Fund regularly comes out for this, but we have of course been here before. Roy Griffiths in effect recommended an independent Board in 1983, only to be thwarted by the self-interest of the mandarins of the time and the hands-on nature of politicians, augmented by the centralizing mission of the Thatcher government.

At the level of resources for services to meet needs, there is in fact a fundamental tension between needs-based generic resource allocation and target-based allocations. Increasingly under New Labour, the latter has come to undermine the former, despite the creation of a new funding formula for allocations to PCTs (2003). As a result, allocations to commissioners for the health needs of their populations are increasingly 'doctored' to suit both national targets and also, now, the local adjustments necessary to allow 'Payment by Results' to work. For example, even an 'under-resourced' area according to the formula may have its budget cuts, if providers are 'over-resourced'.

Resource allocation to health authorities has the advantage of allowing local decisions as to how to produce 'health gain '. Formulae using mortality ratios, direct measures of morbidity and other measures of need are used to allocate resources, and local decisions are possible based on local need. Targets however involve either specific stipulations as to process (e.g. local waiting times) or specific outcomes (e.g. percentage improvements in lives saved in particular clinical areas. They are either applied crudely 'across the board', irrespective of local health profiles, or based on history (e.g. waiting times locally) or are 'rationally' ascribed to each locality based upon that locality's contribution to the national total in line with its health profile.

Only in the last case are targets theoretically compatible with needs-based allocation – and even then, if targets are centrally ascribed, the money might as well as be also, service-by-service. That is, general formulae for allocation and local decision-making are redundant.

If targets involve criteria for expenditure different from needs-based formulae, there will be a tendency for governments to gerrymander allocations i.e. formally subscribe to the formula (which depoliticises spending) yet in practice restrict it or amend it with earmarked allocations. And that of course is exactly what we have seen in recent years in the English NHS. Even after 2003, upwards of 25% of the budget will be for 'central priorities.'

If we have a target-and-league-table-driven NHS, it makes sense to earmark the funds for the key targets. The main problem with earmarking has been that it has been over-applied for trivial sums and under-applied for significant priorities (such as the National Service Frameworks.) The government seeks to have it both ways – by promising less earmarking while mandating more specific achievements. This, again, is through the looking-glass: this gives central government the power to make priorities without the responsibility for implementing them (the 'new devolution' is the oldest trick in the book).

The challenge for the future is to choose either approach – formula-driven resource allocation or 'targets' – and to stick to it coherently and consistently. In 2006, the 'targets' regime has officially been replaced with a 'standards' regime, which somehow embraces national targets, national standards; and local standards. They are inspected by the Healthcare Commission. The dilemma is how to write national 'benchmarks' with local progress. As with schools, do you measure outcome or 1 degree of achievement?

Regarding targets, the main practical challenge is to inject more stability and indeed robustness into the process whereby performance indicators are selectively (and by no means transparently) shaped into the Performance Assessment Framework.

The main problem has in fact been the dissonance between the hundreds of 'high-level' performance indicators eg those chosen each year for the star-ratings or their successor 'bandings' (in 2006); and the monthly, or sometimes weekly or even daily, 'reporting' of the headline indicators i.e. inpatient waiting times, outpatient waiting times, waiting lists, trolley waits; cancelled operations. Boards have difficulty in prioritising, as the political executive does not speak with one voice. It is important that Boards seek to lead and manage 'through' the political jungle, to the benefit of patients and good governance rather than politics. But going against the political grain (eg making redundancies in an election year) may be difficult for service reasons – if, for example, politicians and their 'apparatchiks' do not recognise, at the right time, that 'downsizing' hospitals means investing in the community.

New Providers, New Commissioners?

It is therefore easy to see why the government, sensing the instability of its own central control, sought yet another 'devolving' initiative through Foundation Trusts. But presently there is inconsistency. On the one hand, there is the 'lean, mean' version of the Foundation Hospital, which makes the original 1991 Self-Governing Trust look soft by comparison. This is the version which would dominate the 'new internal market', with a businesslike Board reaching the parts of 'modernisation' that other policies cannot reach. On the other hand, there is the locally-rooted, 'stakeholder'-dominated version, creating a bias towards lowest-common-denominator decision-making. Both versions can be traced to Ministerial speeches.

And what about commissioning? 'Purchasing' was the dog that did not bark for the Conservatives. The Foundation Trust 'policy' paradoxically requires greater central direction of funding flows though larger-scale commissioning – but will this dog be any less hoarse than its 1990s predecessor. Local commissioners will therefore find themselves 'managed', in order to fulfil wider service plans. This is another rationale behind 2005's 'Commissioning a Patient Led NHS', which devolves commissioning to 'GP practices' yet regulates it via larger PCTs. Yet the biggest lacuna in today's NHS, traceable to 1991, is not 'local commissioning' (which is often a red herring in the days of both choice, on the one hand, and clinical networks on the other hand) but what might be termed meso-level planning – below the level of central performance monitoring but above PCT level.

The Foundation Trust should not lead to a divorce from the 'local health economy.' Both NHS Trusts/FTs and PCTs are inter-dependent when it comes both to meeting targets and achieving wider goals. In other words, devolution should not have been about 're-disorganisation' 1991-style, but about freedom from the culture which, despite Ministers' fine words, is increasing in salience – the monitoring culture; the culture in which Chief Executives meet SHAs over every waiting-time breach; and the bidding culture whereby 'kit' and new clinicians are distributed in the wake of Ministerial tours rather than flexible planning.

Different Systems and Clashing Incentives

It is important to choose between different incentive and performance management systems: local collaboration (incorporating the medical professions, unlike the 1974 version); central regulation; central 'command and control' and the various versions of the market. Before 1974, traditional administration excluded the medics. After 1983 but before 1991, there was general management without the market, but even then the corporate management model did not really involve doctors corporately, despite its aspirations. After 1997, local collaboration was the 'Third Way' which replaced the market; but this soon gave way to a mixture of direct command and control and central regulation via fining systems for failure to achieve targets. Yet such targets were often not coordinated with local service level agreements.

Let us consider the 'new market', to be 'rolled out' fully by 2008. The purchaser/provider internal market (1991 version) broke up local cooperation. The new patient choice assumes funding flows which reward choice. But there will still be a 1991-style purchaser/commissioner. Hospitals which underperform will lose income at 'full cost'. But what about hospitals, or specialties and services within hospitals if the system is decentralised, which fulfil their service agreements but cannot meet the demand from patient choice? Will they be 'fined' as a result of lengthening waiting times (through central control) or penalised by losing rank in a new accreditation system? Access to capital may be affected, and a 'vicious circle' of decline may easily set in. In other words patient choice and central regulation may subvert each other. If so, that will produce demoralisation among clinicians and managers as well as perverse incentives.

In the NHS of Sweden and the social insurance system of France, primary care is not central. Patients self-refer to ambulatory specialist care, in the main. Yet the new system in England gives authority over 'patient choice' to the system's gatekeepers – PCTs and GPs. Ministers preach 'choice' without realising it would, if genuinely allowed, sweep aside their cherished 'primary care'.

Performance management was New Labour's replacement for the internal market in the early years. The trouble was that it quickly became performance monitoring by central government – including the development of a blame culture and a 'culture of fear', as meso-level managers sought to 'second-guess' Ministers.

Different policy strands have created unhelpful dissonances. Central policy objectives, with related targets (e.g. cancer policy; the NSFs generally) should be funded on the basis of costed plans, with money allocated to commissioners large enough to embrace clinical networks. Currently, revenue budgets go to PCTs, which may 'sign up' to health economy-wide plans collectively then challenge them individually (or vice versa!). Capital and revenue allocations are less joined up than in 1976, when revenue RAWP and capital RAWP at least led, at Regional level, to attempts to marry the two, imperfect as they were.

PCTs are a problem structurally, and not just because they are 'under-developed' To make rational 'joined up' policy and resource allocations for emergency admissions, elective care and financial balance, there needs to be one organisation seeing the whole picture. Yet even the new PCTs are too small for this. PCTs' therefore 'share services' (e.g. finance; human resources) and also functions. For example, one PCT may 'lead' on emergencies; another on electives' and so on. Solving the scale problem in this way upsets integration; yet having integrated decision-making leads to a problem of scale. As a result, hospitals and NHS Trusts generally may have conflicting demands from a variety of small commissioners. Ironically, as PCTs get larger after 2006, commissioning is being devolved to 'PBC' (Practice-Board Commissioners). Already these GP practice commissioners are merging, as GP fundholders did in the 1990s. As a result, pre-2005-locality commissioners are re-inventing themselves faster than they are being abolished.

One may say, 'that's life', in the market. But such 'life' destroys the NHS's comparative advantage of strategic planning of (on the one hand) complex services and of (on the other hand) effective interfaces between primary and secondary care. If two commissioners in a locality want to support specialised services at the acute Trust and two others want to refer patients elsewhere, neither may get their wish, as the critical mass of provision may result at neither acute location. This is the old 1990s internal market problem, when market forces destabilised services, especially specialised services. Even 'ordinary' secondary services suffer, for providers need to know well in advance where the patient flows will go.

Regional planning's restoration was – rightly – Labour's boast in 1995 (Labour Pary, 1995), repeated in the NHS Plan. It is now a victim of PCT commissioning and the abolition of Regions. Specialised children's services, such as paediatric oncology, require the clear identification of who the providers are, and their clear funding (both capital and revenue.) Yet specialised commissioning is subject to the same anarchy as in the early 1990s.

Conflicting Policy Strands – Practical and Philosophical Dilenamas

Let us review the policies and systems which are in tension? **Firstly**, we have a rejuvenated 'purchaser/provider split', although the phrase itself is unfashionable. 'Shifting the Balance of Power' led to new fiefdoms and jealousies at the local level. The tragedy of the primary care trust (PCT) saga is that both politics and 'path-dependency' prevailed over rationality. As a means of managing and 'sorting out' primary care (i.e. as providers) these Trusts may well make sense. Yet to make them 'commissioners' and trumpet this politically as devolution was a mistake. PCTs' evolution was not based upon a rational or evidence-based approach to designing commissioners of the right scope or size, but was dependent upon the path set by previous policy. Primary Care Groups (PCGs), their predecessor, themselves grew out of the previous (Conservative) government's 'total purchasing pilot' projects. (Smith et al,1996) These in turn had been an ad hoc reaction to the inequities and high transactions costs of GP fundholding. Ironically the wheel has turned full circle, with 'practice-based commissioning' recreating what New Labour spent two years abolishing from 1997 to 1999 – fundholding. Have the transactions costs been forgotten?

Secondly, we have 'patient choice', buttressed by 'payment by results'. If patient choice is real, it will pull the rug from under PCTS, as will payment-by-results, leaving them as cheque-signers rather than commissioners. (And incidentally, even the term 'commissioner' is in most cases a euphemism – purchaser would be more honest.) And if patient choice is 'managed' (as the last government's internal market based on alleged purchaser choice was 'managed'), then patients (or their relatives), GPs, Practice Based Commissioners PCTs and Strategic Health Authorities (SHAs) will spend their collective time seeking to manage and control a highly bureaucratic system, better characterised as the 'new bureaucracy' (Harrison and Smith, 2003) than the 'new market'.

Thirdly, we still have exhortations to – and expectations of – collaboration in local health economies (i.e. roughly the areas covered by the health authorities which were abolished in 2001/2). Yet PCTs have a conflict-of-interest. They are both purchasers and providers. As a result, they have an incentive to fund their own services as fully as possible, while seeking to pay as little as possible to NHS Trusts.

It is widely believed that "primary care trusts have not yet had time to become effective negotiators in their commissioning relations with acute care providers or to develop their planning and purchasing capacity" (Walshe et al, 2004) ie that hospitals outwit PCTs. Yet the real problem is very different. Given that hospital Trusts have no financial margin to speak of and are often expected to classify multi-million pound structural deficits as 'Cost Improvement Programmes', the problem with PCT 'commissioning' is the same as under the last government's internal market – an asymmetry of power and information. Purchasers have the money while providers have the service knowledge. Gaming, and transactions costs, rule (not) OK! Frustration with local haggling is a major source of disillusionment among senior NHS leaders. The mushrooming of commissioning agencies post-2002 has led to a shortage of talent which 'development' can only address so far. And as far as the public are concerned, how can the NHS justify the costs in employing four times as many executives on salaries akin to those in the old health authorities (a fact not unrelated to the shortage just noted).

Furthermore PCTs – even when they seek to club together – are often dysfunctional when it comes to coordinating strategy in order to plan, commission and fund acute and specialised clinical services over increasingly large areas (for reasons of clinical quality, cost-effectiveness and of course the European Working Time Directive). Again, this is the lesson which should have been learned from (less than) a decade ago, when the Conservatives learned firstly that the market had to be managed; secondly that a 'managed market' was an oxymoron; and therefore thirdly that the abolition of the market was not a 'bleeding heart' policy but cold realism applied to a modern public health service.

Fourthly, we have as extensive a central 'target' regime as ever, despite official statements that the number of national targets is sharply reduced. (Crisp, 2004)

It seems that:

(1) there is a basic decision as to whether 'purchaser choice' or patient/GP choice is to predominate. Even after 2008, when allegedly 'full patient choice' will exist, the devil will be in the detail (or, to put it another way, the clash between free choice and 'managed choice' will have to be worked out).

(2) there is a basic choice as to whether the 'market' and choice or central targets will prevail. If a hospital does well and attracts patients with free choice, waiting times may increase, even if only temporarily (this is consistent with survey results showing that – within limits of waiting time – patients prefer quality and convenience to pure waiting time considerations). A hospital may

'win' in the market and 'lose' in the central target/assessment regime

(3) if managed choice (i.e. purchasing) prevails, then there will be a clash between local choice and central targets, as in the 1990s.

(4) local collaboration will be subverted by purchaser/provider splits more than by free choice, as the latter can be modelled by primary and secondary care providers **if** they are acting to aligned incentives or part of the same organisation. Central targets are also more compatible with 'whole health economy' cooperation.

Put whimsically, four conflicting policy regimes are too many, but the NHS could live with two-and-a-half. Why not accept that the PCTs' worthwhile mission was about being small enough to engage with primary practitioners and local populations, in delivering primary healthcare. Making them commissioners too meant setting in train the conflict we now see (pressure to merge, as commissioners, on the one hand; yet GPs seeing them as already remote, on the other.) Service planning and commissioning should be done at a higher level (where the capital is held anyway – another lesson from the last internal market: he who holds the capital calls the revenue tune).

Patient choice is then able to complement rather than supplant rational service design. And performance management can be applied to local health economies rather than individual NHS Trusts and PCTs. And surely that is the overwhelming point about the conflicting policy regimes – they retard integrated care.

Levels of Incompatibility

Mr Blair's two recent health policy advisers evolved two phrases as euphemisms for incompatibilities in policy – 'the balance of fragilities' (Le Grand) and 'constructive discomfort' (Stevens). What these understatements omit is the seriousness of the incompatibility for health services 'on the ground' and also the two different levels of incompatibility – practical and philosophical.

At the **first** level, four conflicting policies create either unclear or perverse incentives. Patient choice may be 'reined in' by commissioner contracts. Commissioner contracting may be reined in by national diktat, regionally transmitted. Hospital developments may be rendered insecure or impossible by 'payment by results' (as with 'PFIs' in early 2006). Collaboration between local health agencies (PCTs and hospitals, principally) may be irritated by both market tensions and organisational fragmentations and jealousies – never mind wider collaboration with agencies outside the NHS.

The more general point is that the government mixes and confuses **regimes** of governance. Along with the 'new governance' (comprising, allegedly, devolution to Foundation Trusts and other agencies responsible for their own 'internal control, yet also – indeed thereby – external control via regulation), we have the 'old governance' of direct political management (sometimes called 'command and control').

It might be better to distinguish command from control. There is indeed confusion as to whether 'command' means an 'order' to achieve outcomes, outputs, levels of activity and other targets, or 'orders' as to how to behave (ie. process). Likewise 'control' can mean either internal or external control (Scrivens, 2005). If the latter, does it become direct management in all but name?

If regimes of inspection, audit, regulation and performance management overlaps and additionally are managed in a fragmented yet fuzzy (overlapping) way by different bodies including government, it is likely to be so.

At the **second** level, we see that basic philosophies of human nature and social behaviour underpinning the four different policies, also clash.

Table 8.1

Social Philosophy	*Policy*
Altruism; cooperation'; 'knightliness'	Collaboration
Workers as 'pawns'	'Command and control'
Providers as knaves	'Purchaser' Markets
Consumers as 'queens'	'Patient Choice' Markets

Even Le Grand (2003) – some of whose language is used above – admits that different 'norms' for steering in public services may be self-fulfilling. (For example the market may accentuate selfish behaviour rather than merely recognise it). As a result, clashing policies based on clashing social philosophies is a serious matter, if anomie and demotivation are to be avoided. Are people intended to cooperate or not? It is not adequate enough to give the glib reply that 'competition can apply in certain circumstances; collaboration in others'. What is at stake here is not business strategy **within** a market, but whether or not a market applies or should apply – and whether market forces are cancelled out by other forces (either through incentives or through the gradual demoralisation of workers).

Additionally, Le Grand's framework of 'motivation' and 'agency' is incomplete and atomised. He lumps together workers and consumers as pawns in the 'first phase' of post-war social policy (the era of assumptions of knightly professionals) but an era of 'command and control' of workers may be perfectly compatible with 'queen-like' consumers. Likewise, empowered workers may co-exist with welfare clients who prefer a passive role.

Likewise an era of professional self-organisation (networks) may also be compatible with active citizens or consumers demonstrating 'agency'. Yet Le Grand's concept of agency is restricted to choice in a market, and his concept of motivation is one-dimensional. All in all, he does not escape the assumptions of 'Modernist Man' so powerfully criticised by Margaret Archer (2000).

What an irony, then, that the one-dimensional caricature, Modernist Man, is the model for the latest of New Labour's 'post-modern' policy strands in public services.

Blair's New Labour: The State of Health?

To return to the beginning of this book, and the title's play on words regarding New Labour's state of health: what does the story of New Labour's health policy tell us about New Labour itself as well as about the likely consequences for the NHS?

Tackling the latter first, there is both an optimistic and a pessimistic scenario. The optimist scenario runs as follows:

The extra expenditure on the NHS begins to bear fruit. Policy contradictions are resolved, with the different policy strands (as just discussed) sees with hindsight to have been chronologically–derived rather than logically–contradictory. Deficits are seen to have been transitory, both a consequence of confused policy pre-2006 and (then) a consequence of further 'shake out' of the system post–2006. Whether it is called a 'market' or 'planning', providers are funded accordingly to their workload and success, in a stable manner.

The pessimistic scenario runs as follows: Despite the extra expenditure on the NHS, the extra healthcare purchased is disappointingly small. The 'four Ps' – pay settlements; 'private deals'; purchasing confusions; and policy conflicts – are both expensive in their own right (ie. 'management costs') and destructive of coherent strategy. New Labour scores a spectacular own goal, at the economic level but more crucially at the political level: it becomes widely believed that 'state healthcare' is a model that has had its day, if it cannot prosper even with so much extra resource. 'Tales of woe' in 2006, leading to hospital deficits and PCTs' denial of care on grounds of 'rationing', become the norm. Satire helps to destroy the NHS ('we can't offer you a bed but we can offer you a 'choice facilitator'). Nothing is as it seems (the rhetoric is of devolution to the local level, yet the reality is Prime Minister Blair deciding hospital consultants' pay rise as in 2006 via a phone-call from Indonesia to Chancellor Brown). Financial problems are 'solved' without analysing their varying causes, and without regard to the inter-dependencies of primary and acute care.

The optimistic scenario depends on 'commissioning' merging with are planning; local health Trusts 'merging horizontally' to integrate primary and acute care, allowing coherent service planning and management; and central government setting overall efficiency targets. Patient choice becomes part of a system embracing a number of social values, rather than an 'initiative' (in the worse sense of New Labour's 'initiative-itis'). Deficits are managed through integrated local health economies, on reasonable timescales (three years rather than one year).

Yet policy confusion may well have rendered the attainment of such very difficult. Part 2 of this book reviewed the **stages** of New Labour's health policy as part of a presentation of its policy-making style in the context of understanding the factors affecting public policy. Part 3 above then reviewed some of the most salient elements of New Labour's health policy, not least in seeking to identify trends and biases as the stages progressed. In other words: is the sheer arbitrariness of the policy strands which emerge from the 'garbage can' diminished somewhat, as we detect a pattern over time? Do more traditional explanatory factors in political science – ideas and ideology; power; political structure (King, 1973; Heidenheimer et al, 1975) – explain how policy comes to 'look' over time (even if it appears as 'garbage' piece by piece)?

The conclusion here is that there is a vision of an integrated, rational approach to policy-making and (therefore) of a coherent NHS, on the part of policy advisors but at a very general level and that it is undermined by persistent tendencies in practice to disaggregation and the 'garbage can' phenomenon on the part of politicians.

Traditional explanations of policy are still important. For example, the centralisation of health policy–making – and of control – in England does give the capacity for rationalisation, if not always rationality, in policy-making. But this structure also, when allied to the culture of the New Labour regime, renders easy the destructive 'initiative-itis' which breeds incoherent policy, and therefore the need for rationalisation in the first place.

It is an unstable mix. Additionally, New Labour has a tendency to construct policy on the basis of image (eg 'community control'; markets) rather than remain open to the counter-intuitive approach which nevertheless makes policy sense (eg the Fordist health service in the post-Fordist political economy). As a result, the rationalisation of the NHS which political economy will necessitate (for the reasons explored in Part 1) may leave the NHS economically balanced yet politically destabilised. Rationalisation will, to the extent it occurs, be in the 'market' direction. But it will not be the socially–optimal market of academic advice. Ironically New Labour will have been bolder than its predecessors. But this may well not be to the benefit of a public NHS.

Bluntly, New Labour may well have bought so much less extra healthcare for its money than it could have, that the social and political forces pushing for increased private financing as well as provision may reach take-off point. In other words, it will have lost the ideological war to defend the NHS (the one war ironically which New Labour shared with Old Labour, at least in terms of tax-funded financing), as a result of policy confusion. Even now, New Labour advisors are setting out the conditions, and institutions, required to make the 'NHS market' work (Stevens, 2006) … while ignoring the corrosive effect of New Labour politics and the culture of policy-making upon these very possibilities.

In terms of this book's analysis of political economy, the NHS may be forced to prioritise 'rational' investment in the health of the more productive members of society, while seeking to keep the middle classes 'on board' through much-reduced waiting-times. But this may be too minimalist a mission to preserve the NHS's legitimacy in the face of disillusionment on the part of those who 'have paid in all their life' and expect care and comfort as well as prevention and quick cure. Likewise, people of all classes may well find the rhetoric of a 'post – Fordist', consumerist NHS at odds with the reality of a slimmed-down, neo-Fordist NHS.

Whether or not this 'state of health' has wider applicability to New Labour's regime overall, is a project of evaluation for others to contribute to, as similar empirical studies of other policy areas, which go beyond the technical, are gradually accumulated.

Meanwhile, the Conclusion, below, incorporates but also goes beyond health to make some observations about the New Labour state.

Conclusion

The New Labour State

New Labour started with the 'ideology of pragmatism' – 'what counts is what works'; policy must be 'joined up'; and objectives and targets set by policy-makers should be 'SMART' – specific, measurable, achievable, realistic and timely. Ironically, this itself is a target which Labour probably wished had been buried by Sir Humphrey Appleby, the fictional Cabinet Secretary who protects politicians from their own amateurish zeal!

Yet recently there has been much understandable frustration on the part of health economists as to the failure of politicians to act on evidence, or to set out consistent ends and seek to realise them. To me, this is evidence of their implicit belief that 'politics' is a bolt-on extra, a kind of nuisance, rather than the basis for understanding why 'rational' approaches of the sort which health economists follow are themselves politically-situated.

We see a benign version of the same in periodic, cyclically-recurring calls for 'politics to be taken out of health' – the underlying implication of the Griffiths Report in 1983 and the Hart report for the King's Fund more than fifteen years later. Yet my response would be the same as Gandhi's response when asked what he thought of Western civilisation – " a good idea, but it will never happen"!

It is not a question of 'should politics feature?' but 'how can we influence politics, through politics, to seek 'rational' ends?' We should not abandon the goal of rationality – either to cynicism or to post-structuralist linguistic nit-picking or post-modernist cultural relativism. But we must unpick it – whose rationality, to meet what ends, with what legitimacy, by what deliberation? These are deep questions, to which technical methodologies can only be applied once the interesting philosophical work has been done (for example, 'Quality Adjusted Life Years' as a means of alleviating healthcare resources only if we agree the ethics and political legitimacy of their foundation; only 'choice' if we know why it is desirable; and so on).

Ironically, the forces of conservatism, that Blair boo-word, have much to offer. Conservatism is the doctrine, sometime justified by recourse either to scepticism and to the human temperament, that that we do not increase human happiness by restlessly overturning established institutions and practices in pursuit of ambitions devised 'rationally' by a well-intentioned elite. Kennedy's Camelot spawned Vietnam, after all. Blair's 'neo-conservative' mentality is the antithesis of European conservatism, whether applied to world affairs or to domestic policy.

And even that is a misunderstanding: the original US 'neo-cons', in the 1950s and 1960s, were former Marxists who became disillusioned with the USSR in particular and moved right in general, skipping liberalism (in the US sense of left-of-centre progressive) in the process. They did not however become boy scouts on the world stage, wishing to contain the USSR, the alleged 'real and present danger' yet eschew global crusading. A contemporary intellectual descendant of the real neo-conservatives – and a respectable conservative in the European sense – is Samuel P. Huntington (1982), known more recently for his 'clash of civilisations' (1996) but (to the surprise of many) a sceptic when it comes to spreading US values in the cloak of universal liberalism, around the globe. Even Francis Fukuyama (1992) cautions against seeking 'the end of history' in rationalistic adventures.

In 1976, Daniel Bell, the sociologist best-known for 'The End of Ideology' (1960), and essentially a real neo-conservative who had journeyed from the far-left without renouncing a belief in social justice and without becoming a liberal imperialist, published 'The Cultural Contradictions of Capitalism" (1976), in which he described himself as a 'socialist in economics, a liberal in politics and a conservative in culture'. If we apply the concept of 'culture' to social institutions such as the NHS, we see why Blair 'simply does not get it' and why breathless 'cultural re-engineering', with its pyrotechnics of (incompatible) initiatives can bleed the patient while seeking to cure him.

Managerialism?

Labour had a honeymoon in opposition with the professions, by opposing the Tory 'centralist state' of the 1990s (Jenkins, 1995) The Tories themselves had been 'managerialist' in the Heath government of the 1970s (albeit of a technocratic, 'French' variety rather than Anglo-American market approach); then increasingly so in the later 1980s under Thatcher (after the first three years, for example when Health Secretary Patrick Jenkin sought devolution in the structure (DHSS, 1981) Perhaps it is easy to oppose managerialism in opposition, as Labour did with its talk of trust rather than contracts in the NHS, which helped its rapprochement in opposition and then honeymoon in government with the British Medical Association. Indeed, given the 'fight for the centre ground' by all three parties in 2006, the Liberal Democrats have identified 'anti-managerialism' in 2006 as a means to oppose both the major parties.

In health, when Labour became New Labour and moved towards the ideology of first 'central control' and then managerialist markets, it replaced its vague 'modernising' aspirations with a harder agenda – and ended its honeymoon with the professions (always unlikely bedfellows – in Old Labour days because of its hostility to private practice; in New Labour days because it identified professions as the 'forces of conservatism').

But managerialism is uninspiring politically. The problem is, New Labour never formed a grounding social ideology. Added to this was New Labour's caution in 1997, with a very timid manifesto. The enthusiasm from the electorate, such as it was, came from the optimism of a new beginning after the tired Tories. The campaign theme song, 'Things can only get better', by D-ream, was strangely apt: it was a new beginning, but from a low starting point – a messianic 'feel' but no prospect of the New Jerusalem. Indeed, this is how it has been. The timidity in actual policy proposals did not matter, at first.

But when the euphoria wore off, real achievement was necessary – both in the search for re-election second and third times around (2005 and 2009/10) and for the 'Blair legacy' (itself a reflexive, post-modern phenomenon – Churchill and Attlee were happy to follow their vision – as they didn't call it – and leave the legacy to the historians, rather than 'storying' it themselves)!

Hence 'public service reform'. But Labour has deepened its schizophrenia here – one strain talks of 'power to the frontline' of the professions, as with Milburn's misleading rhetoric in 2001 (probably self-deluding rather than disingenuous); the other strain characterises these same professions as the 'forces of conservatism.'

There are in essence three normative models for the public services – hierarchy or state control; market relations; and professional self-government. It was the last which Labour seemed to promise in the 1990s in opposition, as the Tories' command state' deepened. (Simon Jenkins (1995) put it very nicely: recalling Bevan's desire to hear every dropped NHS bedpan reverberating in the Palace of Westminster, he pointed out that Mrs. Thatcher's approach was to pick them up, shelve them and number them.) In the Dobson years from 1997 to 1999, the Labour government straddled two horses – trust in altruism (of both the professions and managers) yet also a continuation of the Tories' managerialist reforms in relatively benign form (e.g. Primary Care Groups).

The Milburn reforms of 2001 and, especially, 2002 (see Part 2 above) returned to the managerialist market route, but 'sold' as empowering the professions. This caused more disillusionment and cynicism on the part of doctors than I can recall in the history of the NHS – and also eventual cynicism on the part of the lay non-executives and public involved with the new PCTs, as they found they'd been sold a pup. 'Leadership' programmes for thousands of doctors and hundreds of NHS Boards came to resemble sheep-dips rather than developmental exercises.

So why this counter-productive dissembling? In part, no doubt, cock-up. If we yield to pop psychology, Milburn's control-freak nature perhaps needed to be disguised by the 'smokescreen' of devolution in the NHS (although all the 'devolution' policies were managed down (separate) 'silos' from the Department of Health) – just as Blair's boy scout amateurism in domestic policy needed to be disguised by the rhetoric of 'joined up' policy, to cover up probably the least joined-up policy since 1945.

More significant, however, was the desire to ride two horses – 'trust' and 'managerialism'. 'Trust' implies belief in professional – and managerial – altruism. Unfortunately, New Labour's public service advisers (Le Grand, *op. cit*) came to believe that professions and managers were 'knaves' rather than 'knights' – or that even their knightly motivations needed to be channelled in a corporate direction.

We have seen in Parts 2 and 3 what this did to health policy. Managerialism indeed is the 'new bureaucracy' (Harrison and Smith, 2003) rather than a streamlining of 'corporatist' public services, in which the provider guilds, essentially self-governing professions, come together under state aegis to agree policy-as-compromise. The latter is the German system, which makes the Right's advocacy of Germany as an effective 'managerialist market' public/private mix baffling were it not understandable for what it is – a soundbite to create a benign 'foot in the door' for privatisation, which would look very different in Anglo-American terms.

The new bureaucracy has been a major theme of the New Labour state. Schools, universities, health services…increasingly 'choice' and market rhetoric; increasingly bureaucratic reality. If this is Blair's legacy, it is not even original – it is exactly what the Conservatives left in 1997, and New Labour has deepened the trend, not followed an original strategy…a trend, incidentally, which John Major (2000) regrets when he expresses the wish that he had led a more genuine popular empowerment than his 'Citizens (and Patients) Charters' had achieved.

The new bureaucracy has been accompanied by the very 'Stalinism' which New Labour is so keen to tell the media it has abolished in the NHS, for example, as part of its modernisation. The NHS in its traditional incarnation was anything but 'Stalinist', even in the very whimsical sense that the word is used by those who object to central planning (overtones of Churchill's least fine hour, when he claimed during the 1945 election campaign that an NHS as proposed by Labour would require a 'Gestapo'). It may not always have allocated and used resources to the optimum, but the culture was an open one. In the 1970s health administrators (as they then were) intermittently wrote to the national broadsheets criticising government policy. From the 1980s onwards, that culture changed.

Today, the culture is one of (in the charming US vernacular) 'kiss up; kick down.' Political agendas hamstring local management (eg. no job losses in an election year), passed down the chain of command by intermediary apparatchiks in the Strategic Health Authorities. Then the same local management is blamed for not acting quickly enough to make financial savings, the following year. The rhetoric is of 'communities' and 'empowerment', with 'civil society' replacing the state. Yet local Trust Boards for example, are agents of the state, rather than empowered, or even responsible, actors.

Reducing MRSA rates is aided by lower occupancy and less rush in turnover of patients; yet targets and the financial agenda militate against this and are (most of the time) 'the' deliverables for executives…except when politicians react suddenly (as in March 2005) by announcing that Chief Executives will be personally liable for lowering MRSA rates. (Like Blair's policy of accompanying 'yobs' to cashpoints to fine them on the spot, this one may not apply – but it is the centralist overriding of local leadership and the 'culture of fear' which is the issue.)

In the 1990s, a major political aim of the Conservatives' reforms was to try to devolve responsibility and blame regarding the NHS to 'local management' – 'purchasers' took decisions (whether or not they were the 'champions of the people', as Health Secretary Virginia Bottomley put it in 1992) and 'providers' were self-managing. The public did not 'buy' this, just as Home Secretary Michael Howard revealed the true situation as regards managerial autonomy in the prison service in the famous Newsnight interview on the sacking of Derek Lewis: that is, praise is centralised; blame is devolved.

All modern social institutions require 'managerialism' in some degree. But what New Labour has lost is the concept (and culture) of discretion. Blair was himself ultra-discretionary in his 'policy wheezes', but he led a 'control-freak' government which did not trust the discretion of others – particularly professions **and** managers in the public services. This is, 'market reform' and 'choice' in the NHS turned into its alter-ego – a bossy managerialism.

We see this culture also in education, where the cultural clones of New Labour often have little insight into the nature of their internal reforms. 'The new bureaucracy' is the reality; 'devolution' is the rhetoric. As in the NHS, an overload of central initiatives hamstrings even significant new moneys. Whether in the NHS or in the health services of Africa and Asia, 'devolution' or 'decentralisation' requires both trust in lower tiers and faith in their ability to acquire skills.

Central control and 'the market' are two sides of the same coin, minted in the same language: technical control (by 'top down performance management' or 'market incentives') is necessary to rein in the 'knavish-ness' – or unworldliness – of professionals and managers. Yet it is unworldly of the Blairs and Le Grands (2003) of this world to believe that the market is qualitatively different from state control in steering public services.

New Labour and Political Theory

New Labour is increasingly 'liberal' (i.e. global capitalist) in political economy. In terms of its social and political stance, it combines cultural liberalism (e.g. 'modernisation' of law as regards equality for those of different sexual orientation) with a certain political and social authoritarianism (I do not refer to the recent 'anti-terrorism' and 'identity card' legislation, which stems from special circumstances and should not be glibly absorbed into generalisations.) This authoritarianism applies more in ethos than in law, it must be admitted.

For example, its 'communitarianism' is partly a perfectly liberal demand that people do not adversely affect others by their actions and partly a buck-passing to communities for the local effects of national and international economic forces. 'Social capital' is a very New Labour concept, and typically double-edged – it is 'good' (who's against communities making their whole greater than the sum of their parts) but also useful ideologically to a government which has eschewed overt redistribution to tackle poverty and whose room for manoeuvre on covert redistribution is diminishing (stealth taxes have diminishing returns over time; further large rises in public expenditure will be impossible after 2008 without large tax rises).

Communitarianism is allied with the mantra of 'devolution', of course – 'devolving to localities' is a priority of (what was) the Deputy Prime Minster's department, and a cabinet Minister (Miliband) was appointed in 2005 to work with

Prescott as Minister for Communities. Yet, as with local commissioning in the NHS, 'localities' (intended to be even smaller in local government, with devolution to neighbourhoods and so forth) can be more easily dominated by the special interests and pressures from the arrogant, opinionated and ego-driven than larger decision-making units. The latter have more chance of achieving spatial equity, even if 'small is beautiful' sounds good (Newton, 1980).

Political illiberalism has been shown by the disregard for legitimate minorities (e.g. as with foxhunting) and the placing of political advantage above liberalism ('buying off' otherwise-disillusioned Labour backbenchers and refreshing activists required at election time.) New Labour has sought a 'big tent' in terms of those sectors of society which support it, however passively or even unenthusiastically; but for this to be other than wholly vacuous, it has meant the 'tyranny of the majority' when it comes to issues such as agriculture, the countryside, and development as well as the more emotive single issues such as hunting.

At the end of the day, conservatism (in the European sense) and socialism have this in common: they prioritise the social over the economic in terms of their 'ethic'. In this sense New Labour is capitalist-liberal, and has to attack perfectly respectable alternatives as 'the forces of conservatism' – which is why it is a clever phrase: it can be sold to socialists and social democrats as 'anti-Tory' and to market reformers as 'anti-socialist.' But it is not a Third Way: it is the means by which the 'core constituency' for business (i.e. the Thatcherite political coalition) is augmented is by the sort of interest-group politics which would be very recognisable to George W. Bush, who – like Reagan before him but unlike his father – has run a high-spending, low-tax economy. Thatcher augmented her core constituency by 'ideological' means as well as by this route, it was argued by some in the early 1980s (Hall, 1985). For New Labour, the challenge is post-Thatcherite (ie. accepting the Thatcherite settlement).

Much has been written elsewhere on the nature of this premiership and New Labour Government (Cook, 2003; Seldon, 2004; Toynbee and Walker, 2005, Hyman, *op. cit*). My concern here is whether is there a particular theory of democracy upon which New Labour is subconsciously drawing. In world terms, there is a rather priggish sense of mission – which makes Tony Blair a kinder, gentler, British neo-conservative, on the US model. In domestic politics, there is a schizophrenia as to whether the informed consumer or the active citizen is to be arbiter in welfare services, exemplified by the health issue.

New Labour has a gadfly approach to policy initiatives. As Times journalist Libby Purves put it, 'ministers, desperate for initiatives to feed the media, constantly pull strings without noticing what is happening on the far end. It leads to absurdities: we are promised 'personal fitness trainers' on the NHS, and the Ministry is doubtless wasting money drawing up plans for this. Meanwhile tens of thousands still have no dentist …'.

Another small but notable example is the fact that the Prime Minister did not even know how 'targets' were adversely affecting GP appointments. Mr Blair had an uncomfortable time during the 2005 election campaign, when being questioned by the public moderated by David Dimbleby on Election Question Time: he seemed genuinely taken aback and (in a phrase he has used himself in a populist manner) 'gobsmacked' that the Government target that all should see a GP within 48 hours (presumably, if they wish …) was being implemented rigidly and unimaginatively to suit the convenience of GP practices . Some only take bookings for the day on which it is requested (with the need to ring back if one wants an appointment on another day) and others insist that patients be seen within 48 hours i.e. compulsion rather than preference).

Of course it is quite possible to have fun at any government's expense in terms of the perverse results from well meaning policy. It is important to remember, however, that a kind of 'post-modernist' immediacy, geared to presentation, is endemic to New Labour. Everything is urgent, but also ephemeral. To economically based or 'rational' interests as the basis of policy must be added the effect of 'instant' policy based on a media-filtered reaction to the worldviews and languages of different advocacy groups. Perhaps it would be better to call this post-structuralist rather than post-modern (if we want to have a bit of fun at the expense of academia), on the grounds that – while New Labour is deeply serious about its own 'modernist and modernising' mission (indeed quite po-faced about it) – it nevertheless conceptualises the world, filtered through its focus group approach to defining the political agenda, as composed of different world views based on the different languages of different 'communities'.

Another of New Labour's important themes related to its overall political economy is its denial of the 'old corporatism' satirised in the 1980s, which looking back to the 1960s and 1970s, as 'beer and sandwiches at No. 10'. This corporatism was based on a centralised tri-partism whereby government, employers organisations and trade unions were brought together – most ambitiously, to 'trade off' inflation, employment and the social wage whereby wage restraint would be pursued in return for social benefits for working people.

To some of course, this was and is awful. Liberalism, in such people's eyes, is not about the operation of interest groups, pressure groups and lobbying, let alone institutionalising such centrally in a corporatist state. Yet we should not pretend that democracy and freedom of association can eschew 'interest group politics, whether exercised centrally or locally. Pretending that government represents only the public interest (Lowi, 1995) and not any specific interests is likely to lead to a more inegalitarian society (both economically and politically) than a corporatist society, whatever the practical shortcomings and failures of corporatism British-style in the 1970s.

Academics wedded to the school of 'public choice' and commentators who deplore pressure group activity argue that pressure groups ought to show awareness of the scarcity of resources, and demonstrate how money should be saved in order to afford what they are claiming i.e. to 'make the trade off'. This is an absurdity. In a democratic polity it is the responsibility of the executive (as in the UK) or legislature (as in the US) to make these trade offs and decisions.

New Labour's eschewal of corporatism simply allows a more inegalitarian 'backdoor' influence by elites, occasionally leavened by 'popular consultation' in the public services which changes little. Public choice theory has been responsible for turning the intellectual climate against interest-group politics and corporatism. But 'institutional rational choice' theory shows that 'bureau shaping' may distort public policy even more (Dunleavy, 1991). For example, 'purchaser/provider splits' and provider markets are advocated to diminish the 'capture' of bureaucracies by interests. The 'new regulation' is advocated likewise. But quis custodiet custodes? On this theory the 'self-interest' will distort purchasing, and regulation. Only government can control the 'commissioners', 'purchasers' and regulations. And so we have come full circle. Whoever influences and constitutes government will control the agenda. In the New Labour era, that is international political economy, at one extreme, and the 'garbage can' full of advocates, ideologists and the media, on the other.

What Anthony Downs identified as the inegalitarian theory of democracy (Downs, 1964) – an approach buttressed by the analysis of Olson (1965) and the institutional rational choice theorists of today – seeks to explain activism (or lack of it) in the policy process in terms of costs and benefits to actors. Elites, or those who can achieve concentrated benefits and have means of minimising the costs of mobilisation, are more likely to be active than 'the masses'. Arguments to the contrary in terms of the economies of scale of mass activism still cannot get round the point that benefits to elites are concentrated and disbenefits to the masses are dispersed.

To put it in common language, elites can operate seamlessly behind the scenes, and 'the rest' have to 'huff and puff' and protest (probably to little effect) publicly. It is, ironically, this huffing and puffing which is depicted by New Right theorists as the unacceptable face of 'pressure group politics'. It is inert. Real power is relatively invisible.

It is no exaggeration that, in this environment, New Labour's 'populist initiatives' are both an attempt to 'buy off' its own activists (given its neo-Thatcherite stance on globalisation) and also the urban public with which it identifies. In this context, democracy is defined as 'simple majority rule', possibly overriding the traditional demands of traditionally 'civil' interests. (In other words, pressure is fine as long as we can get away with it!)

One can detect a similarity with the Blairite alignment with aspects of US neo-conservatism. 'Democracy must rule', globally, but it is a thin, or shallow, democracy which cannot be allowed to challenge the dominant regime of political economy and which is defined in terms of individuals as consumers buttressed by 'democracy lite'. On this understanding, 'choice' and 'public consultation' in the NHS are shallow.

The Blairite means of reconciling global capitalism (Price et al, 1999), European Union regulation and domestic policy is to make them as much like each other as possible. Both EU and domestic regulation involve acceptance of markets and the regulatory structure geared to rendering them more competitive rather than restricting them, despite deleterious consequences in areas such as health.

The Final Judgement

Tony Crosland, the leading Labour 'moderniser' of the 1950s and 1960s (Crosland, 1956) once said that Labour was split between radicals and modernisers – that the radicals lived in the past but the modernisers were no longer radical. It seems that today's hyper-modernisers have subconsciously taken that to heart, perhaps with a guilty conscience: they are desperate for their modernising ideas to sound radical.

The trouble is that the New Labour high command is post-modern in its search for radicalism – seeking consumer-friendly 'policy products' on a piecemeal basis, and oblivious to history (even the most recent, as with the likely fate of 'market reform' in the NHS.) By radical, it does not mean a coherent left-of-centre programme which challenges orthodoxy, but the adoption of soundbites and slogans which are chosen to penetrate deep into Tory territory – so much so, that the Conservative leader David Cameron has positioned himself to the left of New Labour, in general but also on specifics such as the PFI in the NHS.

References

Aglietta M. (1979), *The Theory of Capitalist Regulation*, London, New Left Books.

Aglietta, M. (1982), 'World Capitalism in the eighties', *New Left Review* 136, 5-41.

Allison, G. (1971), *Essence of Decision* (Boston: Little, Brown).

Alvarez-Rosete, A. et al. (2005) 'Effect of Diverging Policy Across the NHS', *British Medical Journal* 331, 946-950.

Archer, M. (2000), *Being Human: The Problem of Agency* (Cambridge: Cambridge University Press).

Bacon, R. and Eltis, W. (1976), *Britain's Economic Problem: Too Few Producers* (London: Macmillan).

Bachrach, P. and Baratz, M. (1970), *Power and Poverty* (New York: Oxford University Press).

Bartlett, W. and Le Grand, J. (eds.) (1993), *Quasi-Markets and Social Policy* (London: Macmillan).

Beer, S. (1982), *Britain Against Itself* (Cambridge, Ma.: Harvard University Press).

Bell, D. (1960), *The End of Ideology* (Illinois: Glencoe).

Bell, D. (1976), *The Cultural Contradictions of Capitalism* (New York: Basic).

Benn, T. (1989), *Against the Tide*, (London: Arrow).

Black, D. (1984), *An Anthology of False Antitheses* (London: Nuffield Trust).

Blair , T (1996), '*Stakeholding*' speech.

Blair, T. (1999), *Speech to Labour Party Annual Conference.*

Blair, T. (2000), *Foreword to the NHS Plan* (London: Department of Health).

Braverman, H. (1998), *Labour and Monopoly Capital*, 25th Anniversary Edition (New York: Monthly Review Press).

Burrows, R. and Loader, B. (Eds) (1994), *Towards a Post-Fordism Welfare State?* (London: Routledge).

Cawson, A. (1986) *Corporatism and Political Theory* (Oxford: Basil Blackwell).

Cerny, P. and Evans, M. (1998), *New Labour, Globalization and the Competition State*, Paper presented to the Annual Conference of the Political Studies Association of the UK, Keele University.

Coates, D. and Hay, C. (2000), *'Home and Away? The Political Economy of New Labour'*, Paper presented to the Annual Conference of the Political Studies Association of the UK, LSE and Birkbeck College, London, April.

Cohen, G.A. (1978), *Karl Marx's Theory of History: A Defence* (Oxford: Clarendon Press).

Cohen, M. March J.G. And Olsen, J.P. (1972), 'A garbage can model of rational choice', *Administrative Science Quarterly* 1, 1-25.

Cook, R. (2003), *Point of Departure* (London: Simon and Schuster).

Crenson, M. (1971), *The Un-politics of Air Pollution* (Baltimore: Johns Hopkins Press).

Crosland, C.A.R. (1956), *The Future of Socialism* (London: Cape).

Crisp, N. (2004), *Annual Message* (London: Department of Health).

Crisp, N. (2005), *Commissioning a patient-led NHS* (London: Department of Health).

Dahl, R. (1980), *Dilemmas of Pluralist Democracy* (New Haven: Yale University Press).

Day, P. and Klein, R. (1987), *Accountabilities. Five Public Services* (London: Tavistock).

Department of Health (DoH) (1997), *The New NHS: Modern and Dependable* (London: Department of Health).

Department of Health (2000), *The NHS Plan: A Plan for Investment, A Plan for Reform* (London: Department of Health).

Department of Health (2000), *For the Benefit of Patients: a concordat with the private and voluntary health provider sector* (London: Department of Health).

Department of Health (2001), *Shifting the Balance of Power in the NHS* (London: Department of Health).

Department of Health (2002), *The NHS Plan: Next Steps for Investment, Next Steps for Reform* (London: Department of Health).

Department of Health (2005), *Commissioning a Patient-Led NHS* (London: Department of Health).

Department of Health (2006), *Our Health, Our Care, Our Say* (London: Department of Health).

Department of Health and Social Security (DHSS) (1981), *Patients First* (London: Department of Health and Social Security).

Donaldson, C. and Ruta, D. (2005), 'Should the NHS follow the American way?', *British Medical Journal* 331, 1328-1330.

Dowding, K. (1995), 'Model or Metaphor? A Critical Review of the Policy Network Approach', *Political Studies* XLIII, 136-158.

Dowding, K. (2001), 'There Must Be End to Confusion: Policy Networks ...', *Political Studies* 49, 89-105.

Downs, A. (1964), *An Economic Theory of Democracy* (New York: Harper).

Dunleavy, P. and O'Leary, B. (1982), *Theories of the State* (London: Harvester Wheatsheaf).

Dunleavy, P. (1991), *Democracy, Bureaucracy and Public Choice* (London: Harvester Wheatsheaf).

Dyson, R. (2003), *Why the New NHS will Fail: And What Should Replace It?* (London: Matthew James Publishing).

Eatwell, J. (1982), *Whatever Happened to Britain?* (London: Duckworth).

Exworthy, M. and Halford, A. (eds.) (1999), *Professionals and the New Managerialism in the Public Sector* (Buckingham: Open University Press).

Farrell, J. (2001), *Tip O'Neill and the Democratic Century* (Boston: Little, Brown).

Feachem, R. et al. (2002), 'The NHS versus Kaiser', *British Medical Journal*, January 23.

Flynn, R. (1992), *Structures of Control in Health Management* (London: Routledge).

Foster, A. (2006), Report in *Health Service Journal* of Andrew Foster's resignation remarks, 27th April.

Fukuyama, F. (1992), *The End of History and the Last Man* (London: Hamish Hamilton).

Galbraith, J.K. (1992), *The Culture of Contentment* (London: Sinclair-Stevenson).

Gamble, A. (1981), *Britain in Decline* (London: Macmillan).

Giddens, A. (1998), *The Third Way* (Cambridge: Politics).

Glyn, A. and Sutcliffe, B. (1972), *British Capitalism* (London: Penguin).

Goldsmith, J. (1994), *The Trap* (London: Macmillan).

Goldthorpe, J. et al (1968), *The Affluent Worker* (Cambridge: Cambridge University Press).

Gough, I. (1979), *The Political Economy of the Welfare State* (London: Macmillan).

Gray, J. (1995), *Liberalism* (Buckingham: Open University Press).

Greer, S. (1998), 'Why Won't Companies Reduce their Costs? Universal Health Care and the Flexible Corporation', Paper to the PSA Health Politics Specialist Group Conference, Mansfield College, Oxford, January.

Greer, S. (2004), *Four Way Bet* (London: The Constitution Unit).

Guardian, (2005), p1, 03.12.05 (see also Newsnight (BBC 2), 01.12.05, Newsnight, 14/3/06; Panorama 26/03/06).

Hall, S. (1985), 'Authoritarian Populism: a reply', *New Left Review*, 151: 115-124.

Ham, C. (2004), *Health Policy in Britain* (Basingstoke: Palgrave).

Hann, A. (1995) 'Sharpening up Sabatier', *Politics*, 15, 1 (February) 19-26.

Harrison, S. and Smith, C. (2003), 'Neo-Bureaucracy and Public Management', *Competition and Change* 7:4, 243-254.

Hattersley, R. (1995), *Who Goes Home?* (London: Warner).

Heidenheimer, A. et al. (1975), *Comparing Public Policy* (London: Macmillan).

Hill, M. (1997), *The Policy Process in the Modern State* (London: Harvester Wheatsheaf).

Hirschman, A. (1970), *Exit, Voice and Loyalty* (Cambridge, MA: Harvard University Press).

Hood, C. et al (1999), *Regulation Inside Government: Waste watchers, quality police and sleaze-busters* (Oxford: Oxford University Press).

Huntington, S. (1982), *American Politics: The Promise of Disharmony* (Cambridge, MA, Harvard University Press).

Huntington, S. (1996), *The Clash of Civilisations and the Re-Making of World Order*

(New York: Simon and Schuster).

Hyman, P. (2005), *1 out of 10: from Downing Street Vision to Classroom Reality* (London: Vintage).

James, O. (1995), 'Explaining the Next Steps in the Department of Social Security: the Bureau-Shaping Model of Central State Reorganization', *Political Studies* XLIII, 614-629.

Jenkins, S. (1995), *Accountable to None : The Tory Nationalization of Britain* (London: Hamish Hamilton).

Jessop, B. (1994), in Burrows, R and Loader, B (eds.), *Towards a Post-Fordist Welfare State?* (London: Routledge).

Jessop, B. (1999), 'The Changing Governance of Welfare', *Social Policy and Administration* 33:4, 348-59.

Jessop, B. (2002), *The Future of the Capitalist State* (Cambridge: Polity).

Jessop, B. et al. (eds.) (1994b), *The Politics of Flexibility* (London: Edward Elgar).

John, P. (1999), *Analysing Public Policy* (London: Pinter).

King, A. (1973), Ideas, Institutions and the Policies of Governments, *British Journal of Political Science*, 3.

Kingdon, J. (1984), *Agendas, Alternatives and Public Policies* (Boston: Little, Brown).

Klein, R. (1990), 'The state and the profession: the politics of the double bed', *British Medical Journal* 301, 700-2.

Klein, R. (2002), *The New Politics of the National Health Service* (New York: Prentice Hall).

Labour Party (1992), *Your Good Health* (London: Walworth Road).

Labour Party (1995), *Renewing the NHS* (London: Millbank).

Lea, R. and Mayo, E. (2002), T*he Mutual Health Service* (London: Institute of Directors/New Economics Foundation).

Le Grand, J. (1998) 'The Third Way Begins with CORA', *New Statesman*, 6 March.

Le Grand, J. Mays, N. and Mulligan J. (1999) *Learning from the UK NHS Internal Market* (London: King's Fund).

Le Grand, J. (2003) *Motivation, Agency and Public Policy*, (Oxford: Oxford University Press).

Le Grand, J. (2006), Public Lecture, LSE, London (February 26).

Leys, C. (1999), 'Intellectual Mercenaries and the Public Interest', *Policy and Politics*, 27:4.

Lowi, T. (1964) 'American Business, Public Policy, Case Studies and Political Theory', *World Politics* 16, 677-715.

Lowi, T. (1995), *The End of the Republican Era*, (London: University of Oklahoma Press).

Lukes, S. (1974) *Power: A Radical View* (London: Macmillan).

McLachlan, G. and Maynard, A. (1982), *The Public/Private Mix for Health* (London:

Nuffield Trust).

Major, J. (2000) *John Major, The Autobiography* (London: Harper Collins).

Mann, T. and Ornstein, N. (1995) *Intensive Care: How Congress Shapes Health Policy* (Washington: Brookings).

Marsh, D. (ed.) (1998), *Comparing Policy Networks* (Buckingham: Open University Press).

Mays, N. and Dixon, J. (1996) *Purchaser Plurality in UK Health Care* (London: King's Fund).

Mays, N. et al (eds.) (2001), *The Purchasing of Health Care by Primary Care Organizations* (Buckingham: Open University Press).

Meyer, C. (2005), *DC Confidential* (London: Weidenfeld and Nicolson).

Milburn, A. (2002), *Speech to New Health Network*, January 15.

Moran, M. (1999), *Governing the Health Care State* (Manchester: Manchester University Press).

Navarro, V. (1978), *Class Struggle, The State and Medicine* (London: Martin Robertson).

Newton, K. (1980), 'Is Small Really so Beautiful? Is Big Really so Ugly?', *Political Studies*, XXX:2, 190-206.

Nicholson, D. (2005), Presentation to Foundation Trust 'Diagnostic' Meeting, University Hospital of North Staffordshire, December 21.

O'Connor, J. (1973), *The Fiscal Crisis of the State* (New York: Harper and Row).

Olson, M. (1965), *The Logic of Collective Action* (Cambridge, MA: Harvard University Press).

Osborne, D. and Gaebler, T. (1993), *Reinventing Government* (New York: Plume).

Paton, C. (1990), *U.S. Health Politics: Public Policy and Political Theory* (Aldershot: Avebury).

Paton, C. (1992) *Ethics and Politics* (Aldershot: Avebury).

Paton, C. (1993), 'Devolution and Centralism in the NHS', *Social Policy and Administration*, April-June.

Paton, C. (1995a), 'Contriving Competition', *Health Service Journal*, 105:54465, 30-31.

Paton, C. (1995b), 'Present dangers and future threats: some perverse incentives in the NHS reforms', *British Medical Journal*, 310, 1245-8, May 13.

Paton, C. (1996a), 'The Clinton Plan', in Bailey, C. et al. (eds.) *Developments in American Politics* (London: Macmillan).

Paton, C. (1996b), *Health Policy and Management* (London: Chapman and Hall).

Paton, C. (1997), 'Necessary Conditions for a Socialist Health Service', *Health Care Analysis*, Vol 5 no 3.

Paton, C. et al. (1998), *Competition and Planning in the NHS: The Consequences of the Reforms*, 2nd Edition. (Cheltenham: Stanley Thornes).

Paton, C. (1999a), 'New Labour's Health Policy: The New Healthcare State', in Powell, M. (ed.), *New Labour, New Welfare State*? (Bristol: Policy Press).

Paton, C. (1999b), Commentary on 'Intellectual Mercenaries and the Public Interest',

Policy and Politics, 21:4.

Paton, C. (2000), *World, Class, Britain : Political Economy, Political Theory and Public Policy* (Basingstoke: Macmillan).

Paton, C. et al. (2000), *The Impact of Market Forces on Health Systems: A Review of Evidence in the 15 European Union Member States* (Dublin: European Health Management Association) (for European Commission).

Paton, C. et al. (2001a) *The Impact of the European Union on the Health Systems of Member States* (Dublin: EHMA).

Paton, C. (2001), 'The State in Health: Global Capitalism, Conspiracy, Cock-up and Competitive Change in the NHS', *Public Policy and Administration*, vol 16, no 4 (winter).

Paton, C. (2002), 'Cheques and Checks', in Powell, M. (Ed) *Evaluating New Labour's Welfare Reforms* (Bristol: Policy Press).

Paton, C. (2005), 'The State of Health', in Dawson, S. and Sausman, C. *Future Health Organisations and Systems* (Basingstoke: Palgrave).

Paton, C. (2006a), 'Going Private', *Hospital,* 28; 21.

Paton, C. (2006b), 'Confused policies wrecking the NHS', *Daily Telegraph*, April 5, p2.

Paton, C. (2006c) *Financing, Structuring and Organizing Healthcare Systems* (Keele: CHPM Occasional Paper No. 1).

Paton, C. (2006d), *NHS Confidential*, forthcoming.

Paton, C. (2006e) 'Of Deficits and Reform', Submission to House of Commons elect Committee on Health, May.

Pollock, A.M. (2004), *NHS Plc* (London: Verso).

Poulantzas, N. (1973), *Political Power and Social Classes* (London: New Left Books).

Powell, M. (1999), 'New Labour and the third way in the British NHS', *International Journal of Health Services*, 29:2, 353-70.

Pressman, J. and Wildavsky, A. (1973), *Implementation: How great expectations in Washington are dashed in Oakland,* (Berkeley: California University Press).

Price, D. Pollock, A. and Shaoul, J. (1999), 'How the WTO is shaping domestic policies in healthcare', *Lancet*, 354, Nov 27.

Propper, C. et al (2003), *'Competition and Quality: Evidence from the NHS Internal Market 1991-1996'* (Bristol: Department of Economics).

Propper, C. Burgess, S. and Green, K. (2004), 'Does Competition between hospitals improve the quality of care? Hospital death rates and the NHS internal market', *Journal of Public Economics*, 88:7-8, 1247-82.

Radice, G. (2002), *Friends and Rivals: Crosland, Jenkins and Healey* (London: Little, Brown).

Robinson, R. and le Grand, J. (1994) *Evaluating the NHS Reforms* (London: King's Fund)

Salter, B. (1998), *The Politics of Change in the Health Service* (London: Macmillan).

Saltman, R. et al. (eds.) (2002), *Regulating Entrepreneurial Behaviour in European*

Health Care Systems (Buckingham: Open University Press) for European Observatory.

Schattschneider, E.E. (1960), *The Semi-Sovereign People* (New York: Holt).

Seldon, A. (2004) *Blair* (London: Simon and Schuster).

Smith, J. et al (2005), '*Practice based commissioning: applying the research evidence*', *British Medical Journal*, 331; 1397-1399 (10 December).

Smith, R. et al. (1996), *Total Purchasing* (Oxford: Radcliffe Medical Press).

Stelzer, I. (2006), *The Times*, February 27, p25.

Stevens, S. (2005), 'View from the Bridge: Steering the NHS', Public Lecture to Keele Alumni Association, October 21 (Keele: Centre for Health Planning and Management).

Stevens, S. (2006), Column, *The Health Service Journal*, 27th April.

Stockman, D. (1986), *The Triumph of Politics* (New York: Harper and Row).

Stoker, G. (Ed.) (2000), *The New Politics of British Local Governance* (London: Macmillan).

Taylor-Gooby, P. (1985), *Public Opinion, Ideology and State Welfare* (London: Routledge).

Toynbee, P. and Walker, D. (2005), *Better or Worse? Has Labour Delivered?* (London: Bloomsbury).

Wanless, D. (2002), *Securing Our Future Health: Taking a Long-Term View*. Final Report (London: HM Treasury).

Warner, M. (1994), in Lee K *Health Care Systems: Can They Deliver?* (Keele, Staffordshire: Keele University Press).

Walshe, K. et al (2004) 'Primary Care Trusts', *British Medical Journal*, 7471, 871-2.

Williams, P. (1979), *Hugh Gaitskell* (London: Cape).

WHO (2000), *World Health Report* (Geneva: World Health Organization).

WHO (2006), *World Health Report* (Geneva: World Health Organization).

Index

Abel-Smith, Brian 16
Aglietta, M. 21, 34, 45
Allison, Graham 47, 49, 54, 79
Alvarez-Rosete, A. et al 66
Archer, Margaret 49, 143
autonomy, in rationality model 80

Bachrach, P. 79
Bacon, R. 15, 28
Baratz, M. 79
Bartlett, W. 28, 115
Beckett, Margaret 93–4, 113
Beer, S. 16
Bell, Daniel 33, 148
Benn, T. 37
Beveridge system 30, 39–40
Blair, Tony 8, 9, 86, 120, 152
Blair and New Labour
    conclusions 147–55
    health policy 93–5
    manifesto promises 95–6
    NHS purchaser/provider split abolition
        94, 96
    state of health 144–6
Blunkett, David 29, 93
Bottomley, Virginia 150
Braverman, H. 31, 34
bureaucracy and political bargaining models
    79
Burrows, R. 135
'Butskellism' settlement 16

Cameron, David 8, 9, 155
capitalism
    globalisation implications 21–6
    healthcare system constraints 2–3
    post-Fordism adjustments 15–16
    three phases 28–9
Cawson, A. 47
central control increase 33
centralism
    conflicts 4–6

planning reasons 18–19
    reaffirmation 16
Cerny, P. 27
CHAI (Commission for Healthcare Audit
    and Inspection) *see* Healthcare
    Commission
choice 115–30
    education 115–22
    hospitals 116–17
    PCTs, regulatory role 117
    transaction costs 116
Clarke, Kenneth 122
Coates, D. 27
Cohen, G.A. 46
Cohen, M. 48, 52–3
commissioners and providers 137–8
communication, NHS plan 69
communitarianism concept 32, 151–2
competition state 24, 27
consumer choice *v.* state allocation 116
contented majority phase 29
CORA 32
Crenson, M. 79
crisis
    NHS problem causes 39–42
    origins 16–17
Crisp, N. 141
Crosland, Tony 155

Dahl, R. 79
Day, P. 87
decentralisation shift 105–10
decision-making, public policy implementa-
    tion 79–80
Dobson, Frank 11, 58, 61, 95, 113, 126, 149
doctors' autonomy 40–2
DoH White Paper 2006 60
Dowding, K. 9
Downs, Anthony 154
Dunleavy, P. 79
Dyson, R. 70

For Product Safety Concerns and Information please contact our EU
representative GPSR@taylorandfrancis.com
Taylor & Francis Verlag GmbH, Kaufingerstraße 24, 80331 München, Germany